Vete…
Reflect…

Veterinary Reflections

Contributors
Leonard Black, Mhairi Cameron,
Nicola Gladden, George Grieve,
Andrew Knight and Helen Woodvine

Published by Helen Woodvine

ISBN 978-0-9563633-0-5

A catalogue record for this book is available from the British Library.

Cover designed by Clare Brayshaw

Prepared by:

York Publishing Services Ltd
64 Hallfield Road
Layerthorpe
York YO31 7ZQ
Tel: 01904 431213

Website: www.yps-publishing.co.uk

Contents

About the Authors

George Grieve BVM&S MRCVS

George qualified from the Royal (Dick) School of Veterinary Studies (otherwise known as the Dick Vet) in Edinburgh 1992. He has spent his time since then working in small animal practice. He lives in Ayrshire with his invisible Cocker Spaniel Jasper.

Nicola Gladden BVM&S MRCVS

Nicola graduated from Edinburgh in 2006 and after spending a couple of years in mixed practice in South Wales is now working in mixed practice in the Midlands.

Andrew Knight BVMS MRCVS

London-based veterinary ethicist Andrew Knight has been an animal advocate ever since helping launch Australia's campaign against the live sheep trade to the Middle East, in the early 1990s. He's a Fellow of the Oxford Centre for Animal Ethics; the President of Animals Count: a UK political party for people and animals; the Director of Animal Consultants International, which provides multidisciplinary expertise for animal issues; and the Founder of the Extreme Vegan

Sporting Association, http://www.extremevegansports.org/ which showcases vegan fitness through increasingly novel means of risking life and limb. When not in surgery or at his desk he's likely to be found freezing near the summit of the tallest regional mountain, camera in hand, fervently praying for an audience with the sun.

Leonard Black BVSc, PhD, DVSc, BA(Hons), FRCVS

After qualifying in South Africa (1956), Leonard Black worked for four years in five countries. Eventually he settled in London where he completed a PhD in the faculty of medicine at St. Mary's Hospital Medical School. After several years as lecturer at Liverpool University he took a post as Senior Scientist at The Wellcome Foot and Mouth Disease Vaccine Laboratory, Pirbright but ten years later financial considerations saw the closure of his research department. He and his wife next opened a small animal surgery, starting with a single client on the first day and ending, ten years later, with more than a thousand on the books. Leonard was awarded a second doctorate (1993) for a collection of his research publications, followed by a BA (Hons) degree from the Open University. He won the William Hunting Medal (best paper of the year published in *The Veterinary Record*) and the Univet (Vetoquinole) Literary Award. He played rugby for Western Kenya and was heavyweight boxing champion of his university. He has two adult children and now retired, he enjoys his attractive wife and his own doddering senility in a 17th century cottage near Guildford.

Mhairi Cameron BVMS MRCVS

Mhairi Cameron graduated from Glasgow in 2001. She is 30 years old and lives in Cumbria with her two cats

Noodles and Birkett. She spent four and a half years in mixed practice before moving to solely small animal work. With a real interest in ethics and humanity issues, she loves writing on both veterinary and non-veterinary issues and has had her work published in the local press as well as professional journals. She also enjoys fell running, rock climbing, kayaking and dancing.

Helen Woodvine BVM&S MRCVS

Helen graduated from the Dick Vet in Edinburgh in 2005 and has spent time working in a mixed practice in South Wales. Helen not only has a passion for working with animals but also enjoys sport, particularly badminton and athletics. In her younger days she represented and competed for the county of North Yorkshire in triple jump, 100m hurdles, combined events, cross country and hockey team.

Anonymous Authors MRVCS

A Vet's Mother

One very proud mother who wishes to remain anonymous.

Opening Story – The First Half of The Beginning or the End?

For all newly qualified vets, making the transition from university student to working professional is far from easy. Our first job can be very stressful and the learning curve during our early months (and years) in practice is steep. But, remembering, the challenges for each of us started even earlier, because veterinary medicine is one of the toughest subjects to earn a place for at university. At my interview fifteen students competed for just one place, and many more applicants were not even offered an interview.

Prospective vet students must not only achieve top grades at A level and GSCE, but also have completed varied practical experience with sheep, cattle, pigs, poultry, horses, dogs and cats. We were also expected to spend significant time with a local veterinary surgeon, where we first had to earn our stripes cleaning kennels and making tea! And even at the young age of sixteen, we were advised to visit an abattoir to find out about the meat industry (and also, I think, to see if we could cope with the morbidity we would witness there).

With the need to study so hard and fit in all the practical work experience required, I had little time for very much else as a teenager! However, the vet schools also made it clear that they were looking to take on 'well rounded' students and so they were also interested in extra-curricular activities such as sport and music.

When I first applied to vet school, I had gained a wide range of practical experience as well as the required school grades. I had also achieved in the sports of hockey and athletics and I felt I had a good, strong application. However, competition was very tough and my application was rejected after interview. I can't even begin to explain how desperately disappointed I was, but I was determined – I couldn't imagine doing anything else with my life! Like many of the students who are ultimately accepted to vet school, I had to take an enforced 'year out' before I could apply again. I spent this time gaining yet more experience. But finally I was accepted – I had earned my place to study for the vet's degree.

So the dedication required to be a vet must start from an early age, and the decision to be a vet is one to be taken very seriously. The course lasts for five years, the same as for medicine. After the initial excitement of getting a place and starting the veterinary medicine course, there is, in fact, an immense volume of theory to be learnt, which is broken up by only the odd practical session (where we got to wear white coats and wield a real scalpel, even though our 'patients' were only cadavers!). Even though the academic work was fascinating, the frustration amongst the students during the first three years of intensive theory was evident, as we all craved contact with some real, live animals!

What we may have missed in terms of animal contact, however, was more than compensated for by the friendship and support of fellow students. Vet school functions as a kind of 'large family', as each year group helps those below them. It was a good experience being a part of such a group

– each student had a 'mummy' and a 'daddy' in the year above to help with practical class work. And also a 'kid' from the year below to share your notes with, take out for meals and show around the city. We had our own branded vet school clothing and our own sports teams. The best thing of all was that everyone knew how to have fun, with many well-organised social events, culminating in the 'final year holiday' during which almost everyone in my year enjoyed a well-earned break in Ibiza.

At vet school, some students sailed through the course and some struggled. Many had to repeat exams or even repeat a year – it has been known for the occasional person to take nine years to finish! Unlike other courses, vet school allowed you to repeat a year rather than throwing you out. For some, the study was not worth it and they left the course even as late as the end of fourth year! I too nearly left the course – right at the end of my final year when I discovered that I had to repeat my final exam. I was so disappointed that it felt like a tough decision whether to continue or quit altogether! I am very pleased to say I finished the course and gained my veterinary degree.

As I was nearing the end of the course, I received an out of the blue phone call from a practice I had been to as a student. They offered me my first job. So I was lucky to graduate with a job to go to, and like many other students, I was able to take a few months off to rest before I started work. I spent just short of three years in this 'mixed practice' treating everything from a cow to a hen to a hamster. There was a lot to learn and it felt like I was thrown in at the deep end. My practice offered good support and I soon settled in.

The following stories are written by several vets from across the country. They are a complete mix of happy, sad, emotional and moral events all based on true stories occurring within our busy veterinary careers and reflect the working lifestyle of a vet.

I hope you enjoy the stories...

Eve Gurston

Chapter 1 - Vets' Early Days

Giving Tablets

"Two tablets in one dose, best given on an empty stomach."

Mr Brown scowled across the table at me, picked up the worm tablets, turned and slammed the door as he left my consulting room.

After ten minutes of heated discussion, examination and deep thought I had reached a diagnosis and treatment. As a young graduate, Mr Brown had proved to be my most difficult client to date and hard lessons were to be learnt.

"I usually see Mr Briggs! Where's the boss today?" As a young vet, this was not a great start to any consultation and with a sinking feeling I played my opening gambit.

"Good morning, my name's George. I am the new vet." Things deteriorated with an alacrity that an Olympic sprinter would have been proud of. After much grumbling and expressions of doubt, culminating in "I'll be seeing Mr Briggs about this", I felt totally deflated. The poor Collie sat on the floor, almost looking embarrassed by his owner. 'Mack' had diarrhoea, and had been experiencing the symptoms for almost one week.

"Can you pop Mack on the table please?" The touch paper was lit and the fireworks started. Mr Brown reacted badly to my polite instruction.

"He doesn't like it on the table. Mr Briggs knows that."

This was just the start of the most awkward consultation of my short career so far. I am sure that Mr Brown was trying to make things as difficult as possible. Mack did not go on the table, neither did he have his diet changed to try and alleviate the problem. In fact every suggestion made by the new young vet, was met by 'no' or 'I don't think Mr Briggs would suggest that'.

In those days, I didn't have the people skills necessary to deal with the Mr Browns of the world; college did not equip us for this. Instead, I would become flustered, red in the face and talk much too quickly in an attempt to get the client out the room as fast as possible.

"Two tablets in one dose, best given on an empty stomach." At last I was going to have him out the room and away. A well-earned cup of tea beckoned.

"He'll no take tablets! How am I meant to give him those?" I could not believe it, this was the final straw.

"Just get the tablets into him any way you can, and see Mr Briggs for a check up in one week." He took the tablets and left, finally.

The back door to my consulting room opened and a cup of tea appeared, held by Brenda the receptionist.

"Thanks Brenda. I need that! I hope the boss is enjoying his golf. That man was obnoxious. Mr Briggs does this. Mr Briggs does that. Mr Briggs… That's all I got."

Two days later, my stomach lurched as I overheard a conversation at the desk.

"Half past three Mr Brown, we'll see you then."

"Brenda is that *the* Mr Brown?" I felt sick to my boots, as I knew the answer already.

"Yes. No diarrhoea though, now he's constipated! He's already moaning that it's you and not the boss."

My lunchtime was ruined; I sat in the staff room and brooded over untouched sandwiches. There was no way out of this; I was the only vet to do the appointments this afternoon.

By three o'clock I had managed to keep to time with the appointments, I had no idea what I had said to the clients but things had gone smoothly – the check ups would be interesting! My mind was preoccupied with three-thirty and my appointment with doom.

Grim faced Mr Brown walked in. Mack looked miserable and uncomfortable.

I steeled myself…

"How is Mack?"

Mr Brown looked down at the Collie on the floor.

"I gave him your tablets and now he's not going to the toilet at all." I examined Mack on the floor, just like the boss. The poor collie was very uncomfortable and reluctant to have his tail end examined at all.

"Has he had any bones to eat since you were last in?"

"No bones!" growled Mr Brown. After some coaxing and bribing with biscuits, I eventually managed to get a finger admitted to Mack's rectum.

"You're quite sure about the bones?" The contents of the rectum felt very firm and gritty.

"I know what my own dog has been eating and not eating." The consultation was about to degenerate just like the last one. In an attempt to diffuse the situation I smiled.

"At least there's no more diarrhoea, eh?"

Mr Brown's eyebrows narrowed.

"No bloody wonder with those worm tablets up his arse!"

The penny dropped… I felt both sorry and amused.

The poor dog had had his dignity attacked by Mr Brown's fingers, no wonder he did not want to be examined rectally. At the same time, I was greatly amused. Mr Brown had managed to get the tablets into the dog, just at the wrong end!

Following this episode, Mr Brown will only attend the surgery to see me and we are good friends; I learned to be very careful indeed with the instructions for medicines and to be more tolerant with problem clients.

Mack still does not like to have anyone messing around with his tail end, which I completely understand.

George Grieve

No Rest for the Anxious...

My first year in veterinary practice was somewhat stressful. I graduated in the aftermath of Foot and Mouth disease, which meant that much of my time was taken up with paperwork. I started my first job at a mixed practice with another new graduate and we both got very excited at the prospect of getting to help any 'real' sick animals, rather than just signing movement documents or destroying those poor animals which were suffering as a result of the movement restrictions which were in place.

One exciting day near the start of my career, I saw a total of about ten 'patients' – mainly cattle and sheep. I was beside myself because finally I got to do what I had been trained to do – to fix animals! I worked a long and hard day, concentrating and doing my very best to do a good job.

Later that Friday night, my boyfriend took me out to the cinema. I believe it was to stop me incessantly rabbiting on about all the animals I had saved that day. And he was right, I needed to switch off and relax for a while – we all do after a hard day!

I enjoyed the first half of the film – it was 'Lord of the Rings' – so much that I had forgotten all about 'calving heifers' and 'downer cows' by the interval. Whilst I queued for ice cream, I felt a heavy tap on my shoulder and turned to find myself face to face with an elderly gentleman. He wore an old navy woollen suit and had Brylcreem on his hair. He looked vaguely familiar, I thought. Perhaps he might be a neighbour, but I couldn't quite place him.

"That cow," he said and then paused, staring at me, "she's dead."

"Oh," I replied, at first confused and then starting to feel quite worried, "Sorry, pardon?" I said in a bewildered manner.

"She died," he said, nodding, and then turned to walk away.

My little, new graduate, heart sank. Dead cow. It could only mean one thing – one of the patients from my day's hard work had died. The man seemed very abrupt and images floated through my mind of a complaint being made to my boss. I must have got it wrong somewhere because I thought all the animals I treated that day would survive. Perhaps I'd be sued, in our current litigious climate, or worse, fired! For the life of me, I couldn't remember who this farmer was, and so I didn't know which of my patients had died, when I felt I'd done such a good job all day.

I missed the remainder of Frodo and Sam's journey with the ring, because I was frantically racking my brains to think who the farmer had been. By the time the film ended, I was feeling quite agitated and my boyfriend was dismayed – once again I was obsessing about cows – dead cows now, for that matter. He insisted I didn't go straight into work to check the farm visit book, as I wanted to, and firmly took me home. But eventually, it was too much for me. When my boyfriend started to snore, I sneaked out of the flat and ran down to the surgery in my pyjamas and fluffy slippers, opened up to go inside and scrutinise my clinical notes from that day.

Immediately I let out a sigh of relief, when I realised that the farmer who'd approached me at the cinema was Mr Bowes at Bank End Farm – a tiny hill farm in the 'back of beyond'. I'd been there on a visit the previous day and had written meticulous notes. I had actually told the farmer that the cow was very unlikely to survive and I thought it best to put her to sleep rather than treat her. But Mr Bowes is passionate about his animals and he likes to try his very best to save each and every one. He simply wouldn't hear of having her put to sleep. So I had tried my best for her and then had to leave her in his hands to see if she would pull through. It was one of those occasions I would rather have been wrong, for I really wish I could have saved the cow for Mr Bowes.

Although sad to hear the news about Mr Bowes' cow, I felt enormous relief that it was not one of today's patients who had died despite the good prognosis I had given to each farmer! It seemed that my career was safe for another day!

As I sneaked back to my cosy bed I vowed never to assume the worst in the future until I had all the facts!

Mhairi Cameron

A Dangerous Patient

In the early days of one's career the new veterinary surgeon cannot help but feel apprehensive. Animals come in so many shapes and sizes that in spite of all the years of study, one fears that the next ring of the surgery bell will bring something entirely unexpected.

Only a few months qualified, I took a post in a large animal hospital on the outskirts of Johannesburg. At first everything went well enough and my self-assurance increased by leaps and bounds. However, 'Pride commeth before a fall', and little did I suspect what was in store.

One afternoon a brightly painted circus cage was towed into the hospital grounds and the shutters were removed to reveal a colossal, most ferocious, snarling polar bear. Her drawn-back lips revealed a set of truly terrifying fangs and she glared at us with only one eye because the other was swollen, half closed and infected.

With misgiving I learned that I was to be in charge of her treatment. It was not that I had volunteered for the job and indeed, I would willingly have delegated the task to someone else. However, I was the most junior member of the staff so there was little I could do other than accept with good grace.

Having reassured myself about the soundness of the cage, I decided on a simple plan of action. An assistant was to push a pan of porridge under the bars but hold firmly on to the handle. Then with the bear's attention diverted I was to blow a pipette of antibiotic powder into her eye.

On the first few occasions the plan worked well. Enduring her foetid breath and overcoming my terror at being so close, I managed my allotted task each time and the bear – Miranda was her name – ended up with a good eyeful of powder. However, she snarled furiously and even knowing no bear language, I could guess that she was not trying to say anything really pleasant. On all subsequent occasions, however, whenever she saw me approach with the porridge and powder, she came eagerly forward but anticipating our little trick, she kept her bad eye firmly shut. Although plenty of the powder landed round her eyelids I never again scored a direct hit.

To add to my discomfort word soon got around among the staff and a throng of giggling secretaries and nurses attended each treatment to see us being so thoroughly outwitted.

Whether it was the antibiotic or the passage of time, or perhaps even the porridge that did it, I will never know, but eventually the eye got better and we gathered at the hospital entrance to see the bear off. As the cage drew slowly out of the gates the bear caught sight of me and as usual, she drew back her lips and closed one eye. Most of the onlookers believed that this was some sort of snarl of anger but Miranda and I both understood that she was giving me a farewell smile and wink of triumph. Deflated? … Well perhaps I was a little.

Leonard Black

An Awkward Incident

From the moment the new vet qualifies the public regards him or her as some sort of demi-god who can do no wrong. However, when your halo is knocked askew you return to earth with a shattering bump.

The first two weeks of my new job had gone like a dream. Our practice was in a small Kenyan town, which was surrounded by a vast area of farmland. Everything was exciting for me, a 26-year-old bachelor, and apart from my interesting work there seemed to be an abundance of beautiful women about.

'Make hay while the sun shines' goes the old saying and as this town lay close to the equator the sun shone every day.

I was off duty on my second weekend and was looking forward to a lazy recuperation from the arduous workload. However that was not to be because my boss, being indisposed, asked me to be the racecourse vet on Saturday afternoon in his stead.

"Len," he said, "nothing ever happens there and you need only to put in an appearance." Understandably, I was all too willing to take the extra duty. I had never before set foot on a horse racetrack and rather looked forward to the outing as a new adventure.

I dressed up in my best sports coat and donned my tie with a small horseshoe motif to suggest that I knew a bit about racehorses.

"Half the battle is to look the part," I decided. To finish things off I tied the little diamond-shaped label badge to my lapel, indicating that I was the official racetrack vet.

I felt really important and it was good to be able to drive my car to the stable gates rather than to the public car park like lesser mortals. Although a little late the gates swung respectfully wide as soon as I flashed my official badge. It was all so exciting and new and as I stopped the car my first thought was to make my way to the members' enclosure and sip a cool gin and tonic in the sunshine while watching the activity.

However, I'd no sooner arrived than the loudspeakers blared, "Will the vet please come to the Steward's Office." I was still not too worried as I made my way there, to be told that a horse had been hurt on the far side of the track and could I give it my attention. Expecting nothing more than a tendon injury, I returned to the car and drove round the course. As I passed the grandstand I glanced up and began to feel a stir of uneasiness to see hundreds of pairs of binoculars focused on me.

There was a small group of officials gathered on the track and as I approached, a pathway opened to let me through. It took only a moment for me to see what had happened and to decide on the necessary action. A jagged piece of wood protruded from the railings and the horse must have hit it going at full gallop. The poor animal that lay at my feet had a severely torn abdominal wall and it was obvious that it was almost at its last gasp. The only thing was to despatch the horse as quickly as possible to end its pain and terror.

Every eye turned to me as if to say, "Do something, and do it quickly." Even the big dark eyes of the animal on the ground seemed to look into mine and beg for help. At that moment I wished that the earth could swallow me up because I realised I didn't have a gun with me and only a limited amount of the drug used for the euthanasia of small animals ... nothing in fact that I could use for the present task. I was utterly helpless at the moment when I was expected to do something masterful and to this day I can remember the prickly sensation of the sweat breaking through the skin of my forehead. I must say however, I was not completely to blame for arriving so unprepared. It was the aftermath of the Mau Mau uprising and all privately owned firearms had to be handed in for government storage to prevent them falling into the hands of terrorists.

After what seemed an eternity my guardian angel, who has saved me from countless tight spots during my career, took a hand. Robert, the government vet who later became a good friend, was one of those on hand and, to my great relief, offered to do the job for me using a captive bolt weapon he happened to have in his car.

Feeling very humbled I drove back and, as I passed the grandstand again, the spectators, unaware of what had happened, gave me a big round of applause. I gave them a regal wave of acknowledgement. My heart was not in it but the unworthy thought came to me once more, "Half the battle is to look the part."

Leonard Black

Chapter 2 – Vets' Funny Stories

Wolfie and Henry

Wolfie was an elderly Greyhound who had survived a number of traumas – at thirteen years old he had had a severe fit leaving him unable to stand. After courageously battling through it he was back on his feet two weeks later, albeit with a slightly odd gait. A few months later, he was diagnosed with a malignant skin tumour, but survived another anaesthetic and operation and was given the all clear. A few days after his fourteenth birthday he had a toe removed because of a nailbed infection that would not respond to antibiotics.

But when his owner telephoned me in tears early one November morning I knew that something was seriously wrong. Through the sobs I managed to establish that she wanted Wolfie put to sleep.

He had been wetting in the house, and despite all her efforts including taking him outside every hour and having him checked for medical reasons to explain the incontinence, there had been no improvement at all.

I agreed to visit Wolfie at home as soon as I could to make things as painless as possible for all concerned, and within an hour I arrived with some trepidation at his home. As is often the case, his owner wanted to talk about her decision at some length before we proceeded and insisted on showing me exactly where Wolfie's accidents were occurring.

"I just can't understand it," she wept. "He can still do a normal wee whenever we are in the garden but recently, at least twice a day, I keep finding a puddle just here." She pointed to a pale bleached area on her real wood floor steps. I noticed that Henry, her African Grey parrot, was watching us from his cage above.

I was by this time a little perplexed – it was unlikely to be an incontinence problem if the dog was managing to produce a proper puddle of urine in the same place every time! At that point, Wolfie wandered slowly into the room, sending his owner into another volley of sobs. As I put my arm around her shoulders I was aware in the corner of my eye of Henry shuffling along his perch. He made a sound as though clearing his throat and then piped up as clearly as could be, "Wolfie do wee-wees." In true African Grey fashion his voice was to us, indistinguishable from that of his owner, and it seems that Wolfie was fooled too. Before our eyes he squatted down and urinated exactly where he stood. Wolfie's 'incontinence' problem was revealed to be nothing other than impeccable obedience to his owner's commands, and to his owner's delight Wolfie won a reprieve.

I have no idea to this moment how they resolved the problem and persuaded the parrot to stop leading the dog astray!

Anonymous

Papier Mâché Dog

When I first gave this story to my Mum to read, she thought I must have made it up! But it's true, every word. It was such an unusual case, and Dougal was such a little character, I can remember it very clearly...

Mrs Mckenzie's West Highland White Terrier, Dougal, was quite possibly the most ferocious dog I have ever had the misfortune to meet. On each occasion of my near digit loss, she would look tenderly at the growling white ball of fluff and tell me how impeccably well behaved he was with my boss (who kept booking Dougal in to see me because he was terrified of the dog!).

"Oh, but he's such an angel with Dr Jackson," she would repeat over and over. Apparently his 'Tasmanian Devil-like' behaviour was reserved just for me!

So, you can imagine my amusement when the practice received the call from a very distressed Mrs Mckenzie reporting that Dougal's mouth had been 'glued together' after his usual breakfast on the morning post. My nurses couldn't quite understand what the distressed owner was trying to tell them, so, after two of them had tried to make sense of Mrs Mckenzie, they handed the phone to me with an incomprehensible look.

At first, I couldn't quite believe my ears, but Mrs Mckenzie sounded very upset, so I told her to bring Dougal in to see me immediately.

About 10 minutes later, she presented me with one very, very angry Westie. If he were human, his face would have been scarlet and there would have been steam blowing from each ear! Poor Dougal, indeed, couldn't open his mouth an inch. Try as he might to bite me, the best he could manage was an angry poke with his cold wet nose, and a severe glare for good measure!

It was very hard not to laugh, because I realised this wasn't a serious condition – even though I had never seen anything like it before. For the first time ever, I was able to lift Dougal's lips and examine the razor sharp 'tools of terror' beneath.

"Hmm, he's got a good set of gnashers there," I commented, making a mental note to be even more careful to steer clear of them in the future! Dougal's 'gnashers' were completely embedded in what can only be described as partially set papier mâché. He forcefully exhaled spit and little missiles of paper with each breath, which smudged on my glasses and face. But try as he might, he couldn't wrench open his jaw to bite me. This seemed to distress Mrs Mckenzie no end, and she patted and reassured him after each and every attempted snap!

We admitted Dougal immediately for a general anaesthetic to allow us to scrape the mâché off his teeth. This was rather a long-winded procedure as the glue from the envelopes he had chewed had hardened the paper considerably. Finally we were able to prise Dougal's jaws apart and remove the rest of the paper. On some of the larger pieces, I noticed odd words and figures. I think it was a council tax bill, so I made sure to tell Mrs Mckenzie later so she could request a further copy from the council!

As soon as we removed the breathing tube from Dougal's windpipe, he started snapping and growling – before he was even properly awake! He made a speedy recovery and Mrs Mckenzie was beside herself with joy when we asked her to come through and retrieve her dog from the kennel. He had chewed through the lead we had attached to him to pull him gently but firmly out of the kennel without having to get too close (a technique we must often employ with very dangerous dogs to maintain staff safety). As soon as Dougal saw his 'Mum' however, he yipped excitedly and jumped up into her arms, looking like butter wouldn't melt.

Mrs Mckenzie brought us a large box of chocolates to say thank-you, and Dougal said thank-you in his own way, three weeks later, when he nipped my boss on the bum whilst he bent down to get Dougal's annual vaccination out of the fridge!!

Mhairi Cameron

Poison...

Calves on the farms were sometimes taken by prowling leopard and although I never saw one I often had to treat dogs poisoned by the strychnine used in leopard bait. The lethal effects of this poison are due to respiratory failure and caused by severe muscle spasms. Simply relaxing the victim by anaesthetising them for a day or two was generally an effective treatment.

Snakebites in dogs were also common because in the hottest part of the year snakes, mainly puff adders, were common and walked about arm in arm as if they were the master race. They could be seen on almost every journey sunbathing on the dusty roads and it was easy to imagine a smile of sheer bliss on their reptilian features. I often think that the enjoyment of sunshine must be even greater in cold-blooded than in warm-blooded creatures like us.

Dogs bitten by snakes could sometimes be saved from the poison's immediate effects but recovery was complicated because a large area of tissue surrounding the bites usually sloughed away, making healing slow.

People were usually bitten when these lethargic reptiles were inadvertently trodden under foot. However adders do not rear up so wearing gumboots generally ensures safety.

When the wet season comes to Kenya the heavens open and the rain pours down in a way that cannot be described to those unfamiliar with African conditions. Mud is everywhere and according to custom, muddy boots are left outside the kitchen door in the evenings when, tired out, you reach the warmth and comfort of a dry farmhouse.

One lovely morning I raced out after breakfast, late as usual and without a second thought thrust my foot into a boot, only to find it already occupied by something cold, slimy and alive. In that instant I must have aged by ten years and in abject terror, kicked off the boot. The boot flew in one direction and a fat bullfrog flew in the other!

The lesson is well learned. Although I now live in Surrey where the puff adders are few, I still check my shoes carefully every morning before putting them on.

Leonard Black

Sheepish

When the telephone went at four-thirty in the morning it had to be a 'proper' call, not just an enquiry...or a lost cat. My heart sank when I heard the farmer's voice; I was a small animal vet working in a mixed practice, the chances of being called out by a farmer were remote – that's what they'd said at the interview anyway.

"She's pushed her lamb bed out, can you come straight out?" I looked at the clock, 4.45am – why didn't farmers work 'proper' hours?

"Yes John, be there in twenty minutes." I knew the farmer and his farm's location, which was a bonus. A lamb bed is a local expression here for a prolapsed uterus – a condition whereby after lambing the ewe continues to push and forces her uterus to involute, that is to turn itself inside out and prolapse out of her vulva to the outside world, leaving it hanging from her rear end and trailing behind her. This is a serious condition because if it is not replaced as soon as possible the uterus will swell and increase in size. The tissue will get covered in dirt and bacteria, and will eventually start to become necrotic (die off). If the prolapse is not replaced the ewe could die from the shock that is induced. Indeed she needed attention straight away.

After ten minutes I was at the farm. The farmer in question was known within the practice for his lack of patience and his lack of humour, this was a very awkward call.

"How long has it been out John?"

"Probably most of the night, I checked them at midnight and went to bed. They were OK then."

"Can you grab her; I'll go and get my kit." I set off for the car, a prolapsed womb in a sheep was easy, even for a small animal vet like me, and I'd be back to bed within an hour. All I had to do was give her an anaesthetic nerve block to alleviate her discomfort and attempts to push against me, clean up the uterus, replace it and stitch round her vulva to keep it in. Simple.

But two hours later, I was still at it. The conversation had been fine for the first forty minutes, after that, things had kind of dried up, I should have been finished and John knew it; it wouldn't be long before he started to get grumpy.

The prolapse was swollen as it had been out for most of the night and the uterus was now twice the size it should be. I had given her steroids to try and reduce the swelling but it was awkward trying to get the enlarged organ back through the hole it had come out of. I succeeded several times in replacing the organ but no sooner had I pushed the prolapse back in, she gave one almighty heave and pushed it straight back out again. As if that wasn't bad enough she then struggled to get back on her feet. John quickly helped me keep her still, whilst I had yet another attempt. I had administered an epidural (anaesthetic nerve block) to freeze the area, but she was still managing to struggle and persisted in pushing against my continuous efforts to force the swollen uterus back in. Time was passing quickly as the prolapse refused to stay in and I felt every minute of it. I swore under my breath and I hoped that John would not lose his patience.

John's wife came out with tea, a grim look on her face.

"She'll be for the knacker after all that plestering about." I cringed at her comment as I replaced the uterus back inside the ewe. To my relief, this time it stayed in – no struggling, no kicking or thrashing at all. I quickly stitched the vulva, holding the prolapse in but leaving enough space for the sheep to pass urine. The job was done – it couldn't possibly come back out.

"That was a tough one, John."

A glimmer of a smile played across the farmer's face.

"That'll dae her! Are ye staying fir breakfast?"

"No thanks, I'll get back home and walk the dogs." I was tired and wanted to wind down by walking my dogs before I had to be at the surgery for the morning consults. I gathered up the gear and the dreaded emergency telephone and made a getaway.

As I drew up at the house the telephone went. The patron saint of vets-on-call was not smiling today.

"Hello, how can I help you?" I had my eyes shut, and my heart had accelerated to the speed of a runaway train.

"Please make it a lost cat!" I thought to myself.

"George? It's John here!"

I almost collapsed onto the steering wheel; the prolapse must have popped out again…I felt devastated. I didn't wait to hear anything more.

"I'll be back in ten minutes John."

"Dinnae bother – she's deid!"

"Dead?" My heart plummeted through my shoes and through the floor of the car. All that work, for nothing! There would be the inquest with the boss, and the farmer would be let off with the bill – I felt devastated.

"Aye she's deid, drooned herself in the water trough! Her lamb bed is still in though. I jist thought ye'd like to know. Thanks anyway! See ye next time." The telephone went dead. I sat for a moment and digested the news, and then I started to giggle. Rather than face the embarrassment of being fixed, the sheep had done the only thing a proper sheep could do and had drowned herself in the water trough! There must be easier ways to make a living!

George Grieve

'Eefer' Bloke

I set off from the practice, with directions to one of our farm clients, Mr Jones. When I had asked for directions, the ex-partner of the practice had laughed and said "Ahh, Mr Jones, our brightest client!" Being quite new to the practice, I had not met our entire client database yet and I wondered what was in store.

The piece of paper that Joan, the practice manager, had scribbled directions on for me said I had to turn 'left, left again, then right, and continue down a narrow track to find a small farm which straddles the road'. Apparently there 'in the middle of the yard' would be this '1950's style tall feller'. It sounded like he was such a permanent fixture, there in the middle of the yard, that he should be displayed on an Ordnance Survey map!

The journey was not long but after crossing an A road my route became narrow with few passing places. It was a hot summer's day and many of the hedges were overgrown. There were no grass verges and I could not see over the hedge. It was like driving through a tunnel and such a shame that I could not enjoy the nice view that was on the other side. Perhaps one day I would be able to afford a four-wheel drive where I could sit higher up and see over the hedges. Then I would be able to admire the glorious countryside that I knew existed, at a slow speed, just like the farmers do in their Land Rovers in the early hours of the morning. At one point the road was so narrow that I could hear the sharp branches of the hedge putting fine scratches down each side of my car. I could never understand why the council only allowed so few passes of hedge cutting as it allowed the hedges to look scruffy and untidy. I had the windows down as my air conditioning had packed in and when there was space I hung my arm out of the window to catch the passing air, sending a draft up the inside of my T-shirt to cool me down. There were many unsignposted roads especially in the narrow network of roads linking the small villages deep in the Welsh countryside and it was all too easy to get lost, driving oneself round in circles. On the map it was not possible to tell which were junctions and which were through roads and I had a lot of fun in the first six months trying to find my way around the new area. I also had the added problem that I could not pronounce any of the villages on the map, which caused me a few problems a time or two when clients could not work out where I was when I got lost and I had to get them to spell out the names every time. I am pleased to say though I have greatly improved in my ability to read the Welsh place names since working here.

My directions this time were quite simple and I had been given plenty of landmarks (usually in relation to a pub!). As I drove down the lane, I looked for the farm. It was not difficult to find, as it was the first one I came to with buildings on both sides of the lane but I continued to drive past wondering if this was the right place. To my surprise, as I drove past the first set of buildings, I saw to my left a tall man in a long black duffel coat, fastened with orange baler twine round his waist. Beneath this, he wore a blue boiler suit and I noted several jumper collars around his thin neck. He had thick black-rimmed glasses, straight from the nineteen fifties, with bushy dark eyebrows jutting over the top. His black hair, now heavily flecked with grey, escaped untidily from under his flat cap. He just stood there, statue like, in the middle of the small concrete yard, staring vacantly into space and he was, I thought, somewhat inappropriately dressed for such a hot summer's day!

I chuckled to myself as I realised I must be in the right place as the description fitted exactly. I couldn't believe he was standing there just as it was written into my directions. So I stopped my car and reversed into the yard where he was standing. I turned my paper with the directions over so it was not possible to read the description should anyone look into the car. The man didn't move.

As there were a lot of farmers with the surname of Jones in the area, and I wanted to double check that I was in the right place, I could hardly just say "Mr Jones?" I couldn't remember the farm name nor pronounce it so I decided to check that he was having a pre-movement TB test.

"Have you got some cows to pre-movement test?" I asked.

Silence. He didn't even twitch.

So I said, "Am I at the right place, I've come to do a TB test?"

Silence again. At this point I wanted to wave my hand up and down in front of his face to see if he was actually alive! However, I managed to refrain. Why he was rooted to the spot I couldn't figure out.

"Eefers," he spoke finally.

"Pardon?" He was quietly spoken and his accent was so strong that I failed completely to understand him.

"Eefers," he repeated, just as cryptically as before. I racked my brain, hoping for some kind of understanding

… 'Eefers' … 'Eefers' … I thought … Oh! 'HEIFERS'! My brain clicked finally. A heifer is a young, female cow before she has given birth for the first time.

"Have you made a list of the ear tag numbers already or would you like me to write them down as they go through the crush?" I asked, feeling very pleased with myself for getting over the first communication hurdle.

Silence. Does HE understand ME, I wondered. I know my accent is also strong and I'm not from round here, but I didn't know what else to say to him.

"Wife," he replied in a grunt, nodding his head imperceptibly towards the farmhouse. I looked around, just in time to see a smaller woman wearing a moth-eaten green jumper appearing from behind a rotten wooden door. Her back was rounded as she hurried attentively down the path towards us.

At this point Mr Jones finally started to move and we all crossed the road to where there was a crush set up ready and waiting. The 'wife' went to the front of the crush, standing a metre or so away from the door. Mr Jones disappeared inside the shed amongst his cattle, followed by his son who suddenly appeared from nowhere. The shed was very small and old fashioned, built of stone with a low slate roof, which would hardly keep much rain out. It was a far cry from the modern farm buildings today of steel frames, Yorkshire boarding and concrete sides which house hundreds of cattle and can be mucked out by machine. Mr Jones must spend many hours hand-forking manure and barrowing it out of the shed. The entrance was a standard door size and Mr Jones' son had parked the crush just outside the doorway. Normally this set up is the most awkward to get cattle into a crush as there is no race and instead farmers spend time chasing the cattle in circles, never thinking to use a few gates to help funnel them in. There were no sticks used to get the cattle into the crush, as other farmers would have done, instead Mr Jones pushed each cow individually by putting his body and arms round its rear end and holding on to either side of the crush. He made the odd glance in my direction and smiled stupidly, still not saying anything. When he smiled I could see he had some teeth missing and those he had left had a black rim round each tooth near his gums. Slowly but surely he managed to get each cow into the crush without any swearing or sweating or even breaking into a run.

My clippers broke the uncomfortable silence for a short time, followed by the click of my TB injection guns. I wrote the ear tag number down before opening the crush door to release the first heifer. She ran out at speed, braking suddenly, almost running into the 'wife', who stood rooted to the spot, and turned sharp left and into a field, before disappearing out of sight. Mrs Jones didn't even flinch! It's a brave woman that stands her ground when a cow runs at you! It could have slipped and rugby tackled her!

The three Jones' worked well together with hardly an exchange of words. I thought to myself – are they psychic? It was almost surreal how they all moved around so quietly in silent communication. What little was said was in Welsh, I think that genuinely they struggled to speak any English. Perhaps that was why he had taken so long to respond to my questions. Most of the farmers that normally spoke Welsh were fluent in English, though many were rude by only speaking English to ask me a question and chatting to each other in Welsh so I could not be included in the conversation.

Next we crossed the yard and went into an old cow byre where he had already chained up a couple more cows ready for me to test. The chains were round their necks to keep them next to a concrete division so I could walk between each cow individually without her walking off. Cow byres like this are now more of a rarity as most modern farms now have new style herringbone parlours to milk their cows and new cubicles for them to lie in. Although now beef, this farm must have had a milking herd years ago. The cows were contentedly eating some cake and they did not notice the jab of TB I gave them. Mr Jones smiled and stroked each cow, proud of her condition and temperament.

After I finished the test, I was invited inside to wash my hands. I made the mistake of taking my wellies off! I tried to pick my way over a dirty, dusty concrete floor with sharp splinters sticking to my socks. When I got to the sink I was able to take my eyes off my feet and look around the room – is this an outhouse, I wondered? Surely it can't be their home! But there was a sofa, well, after a fashion, if you ignored the dust and covers. Wait – was that a cooker? I could just about make out the ring from under a black pan. Surely not! The actual house must be through the door in the corner, perhaps this is a porch. I couldn't look round for too long as Mr Jones followed me in.

I quickly washed my hands and returned outside. As I packed my equipment away I looked around; the house, the buildings, the little old tractor – you would never have thought this was the 21st century.

It turned out that when I read the test three days later that one of the cows had failed the test and was to be slaughtered. I tried my best to explain that they were now on restriction and that they could not sell any animals. He vaguely nodded so I thought I had got through. I did not have any paperwork with me to give him at the time to officially serve the restriction. As I drove away I decided to ask my boss if it would be acceptable to post it to him or whether I should get one from the surgery and drive back.

"Who is it?" asked the boss.

"Mr. Jones," I said.

"Which one? There's hundreds!"

"The skinny one that doesn't say anything with the duffel coat! The nineteen fifties style statue," I replied.

"Oh him, bloody hell. No, you'd better drive back, he's not the brightest, he won't understand a thing."

Tired after a long day, I quickly collected the form and sped back to the farm. The journey this time seemed shorter as I now knew my way. I knocked on the door – no reply. So, boldly, I tried the door. It was not locked and with a loud crack as the wood suddenly became unstuck, it opened and I poked my head round. There they all were sat on the 'sofa' not saying anything making me feel a little rude for blundering in. So this IS a house I thought!

"Oh hello. I just have to give you this form to say that you can't sell anything, I'm afraid," I said, holding up the form and pointing.

"Can I sell the other four then?"

"No, you're on a movement restriction now."

"But can I sell them?"

"No you can't sell anything at the moment."

"So when can I sell them?"

"Well you'll need a retest first which you'll have to pass."

At this point I felt like giving up but he seemed satisfied with my answer, or else he gave up on my accent!

Since then I have been back to Mr Jones' farm again, he now has a little more to say because he has seen me before. I don't know if they ever actually leave the farm, but he would be easily recognisable if they did. He is a gentle farmer who lives in his own little world, doesn't go anywhere or change his clothes – having no money to do so. He doesn't shout or lose his temper and brings his cattle in by leading the way with hay. He only keeps a few cows and with the state of today's agriculture I do not know how he manages to earn a living. He keeps beef cows and whilst normally renowned for being wild and dangerous, his are all quiet, making them more pleasant to work with. His only tractor is an old Ford 3000 which the son moves the short distance from its place in the yard to position the crush. You can see his brain working – turn the key, foot down on clutch, move gear stick, lift the back arms, foot up off the clutch. It always takes him some time to set off.

I must say, however, that I like going to this farm for my memories of that first visit, and the knowledge that they are all completely harmless, and they never say anything so I don't even have to talk about how bad the weather is or whether TB is increasing, or the price of beef. I am currently the only member of staff privileged enough to have washed my hands in the house! Now, I even get a bucket of hot water, soap and a towel brought to me!

I have never seen another farmer living in such conditions since, but it makes a lovely change to see a farmer who genuinely likes to keep his animals and is happy with what he has got. I have seen him leading his small herd inside with nothing but a slice of hay, feeding the leading cow with the odd mouthful to keep it coming, and also gently stroking his cows – and I know it's not just to keep them quiet for me to work on.

Anonymous

Chapter 3 - Vets' Morals and Frustrations

The Hazards of Giant Stomachs

It was supposed to be a nice, easy morning at my new hospital.

"Just a couple of spays and castrations," the other vet smiled reassuringly. "We thought we'd ease you in gently," she offered, as I tried to disguise my relief. Having endured one of my most hellish weekends at this hospital previously, I was well aware of its reputation for unexpected emergencies. It was, therefore, with no small degree of trepidation that I had accepted an offer to relieve the second vet for the week. Locum vets must, however, go where the work is.

I unsuccessfully attempted to locate a hospital coat as my colleague steered me around the hospital in a flurry of distracted conversation. Given their propensity for accruing animal hair, pus, blood and other noxious substances, I had learnt to avoid using my personal coats wherever possible. The place still appeared to resemble the maze of corridors and stairs I dimly recalled, and by the time the first patients and their guardians started to fill the waiting room, the available drugs and equipment, the names of the staff and their roles, and the hospital protocols, if any, remained shrouded in mystery. Thankfully, I would have plenty of time to settle in, or so I thought.

Things were soon looking up. I was operating rather than consulting, and while my colleague saw the first patients I managed to locate not only a coat to protect my clothes, but even the hospital stash of instant coffee – cunningly hidden in the depths of a cupboard! The nurses were thrilled when I offered them a hot drink. "A vet who makes coffee!" often seems to be a rare species, reflecting, perhaps, an inexcusable degree of arrogance, or thoughtlessness, among too many veterinarians.

Steaming liquid sustenance was soon distributed, which was followed in short order by the arrival of one scruffy, wire-haired and very enthusiastic puppy, and a moderately anxious black and white feline. Both were examined and duly admitted for their routine neutering operations. As I relaxed and started to calculate their drug doses a phone rang urgently somewhere in the background. My heart sank as a muffled conversation complete with expletives in the unmistakable accent of my erstwhile colleague drifted down the corridor, followed soon after by the ominous tread of her footsteps.

It transpired that one of our satellite branches had just seen a very, very large dog, with depression and a slightly bloated abdomen. In short, they suspected gastric dilation-volvulus, or 'twisted stomach,' which large breeds are prone to. They had sent the dog to us, claiming – probably correctly, as it turned out – that their facilities were not large enough to house it!

In such dogs the considerable weight of a heavy meal, especially if followed by exercise, can actually cause the stomach to twist. This blocks the stomach outflow, which can result in a steady expansion as the contents ferment, producing gas. The pressure of the expanding stomach soon exceeds that in the neighbouring veins, thereby blocking the return of blood from the lower half of the body to the heart – and thereafter, the rest of the circulation. The result is plummeting blood pressure, shock, collapse and death, usually in rapid succession.

Emergency surgery is required, during which the stomach is decompressed, un-twisted, and anchored to the abdominal wall, to prevent recurrence. The technique was beautifully described in the illustrated small animal abdominal surgical manual I had foolishly left at home, thinking that I would only be there for a week, and that my technical library was far too heavy to lug around. A quick check confirmed my worst fears: this so-called 'hospital' lacked a soft-tissue surgical text. Unfortunately, I had not yet seen such a case in five years of practice, and it remained the last major soft-tissue surgery I was unsure how to perform. I knew I had been very lucky to date, and that my luck was bound to run out someday.

Half an hour later the dog duly arrived. At 83.5 kg, she was the largest animal I had ever treated, other than one very fat Rottweiler requiring a blood test, with jugular veins buried beneath layers of fat. Suzie on the other hand, was an Irish Wolfhound – the world's largest breed – and fairly lean. This was, however, somewhat disguised by what appeared to be an ominous swelling of her abdomen. My valiant attempts to feel the contents of this enormous, firm abdomen were rapidly revealed to be futile, and so we proceeded quickly to the X-ray room, after taking blood samples for in-house analysis.

Although her legs protruded far beyond its edges, we somehow managed to balance Suzie on the X-ray table. Incredibly, she tolerated our manipulations with quiet grace. Thankfully, it appeared sedation would not be required. The machine itself was less cooperative, however.

Our largest X-ray plate would reveal only around a third of Suzie's abdomen. However, by piecing together different views, I confirmed that her intestines had been pushed towards her tail by a massive, gas-filled organ in the front of her abdomen – doubtless her stomach.

Although almost the largest dog I had ever seen, the magnanimity of her spirit appeared to match Suzie's size. She lay calmly and quietly, eyes always upon us, as we manipulated her into awkward positions. I felt safe putting my face only inches from her jaws, as I applied my stethoscope repeatedly to her chest. Her heart rate and breathing were steadily climbing – sure signs of progressing shock.

Fortunately, Suzie's owners had had the foresight to invest in pet insurance, and so were able to afford the £2,000+ bill the X-rays, blood tests and surgery would eventually necessitate. They had already provided consent for surgery if necessary, and so without further delay we walked Suzie into theatre. We rapidly connected both arms to fluids set at maximal flow rates, to try to counter her shock; induced anaesthesia, and prepared her for surgery.

In Suzie's case an appropriately sized incision ended up nearly 30 cm long! Experienced from countless spay operations, I had no trouble entering her abdomen, whereupon I soon discovered the largest stomach I had ever seen. At around 30 x 20 x 15 cm, it appeared to be distended with gas – conclusively confirming the diagnosis of life threatening stomach dilation. Oddly, the stomach did not appear to be twisted, even when I inserted my arm up to the elbow, feeling the outside of it all the way to the stomach outlet.

I was fast approaching the limits of my surgical experience, when my colleague arrived to assist. Fortunately, with 10 years of experience, she had dealt with several such cases. She first passed a stomach tube via the mouth, to decompress the stomach. Although I could feel the tube with my hand, confirming its location, the stomach stubbornly refused to decompress. We eventually succeeded by puncturing it with large sterile needles, which resulted in the whistling exodus of foul-smelling gas. My colleague was thereby able to confirm that the stomach contents had begun to ferment. Rather than creating a free gas pocket, this had resulted in a 'frothy bloat,' which is much harder to expel. However, by lavaging the stomach with warm water passed via the stomach tube, we were able to empty it of Suzie's last meal, as well as a considerable quantity of fluid and gas. Finally, we flushed it with activated charcoal solution, to help remove any remaining chemically active compounds.

Whilst squeezing out the stomach contents, I detected something firm at the stomach outlet. About three inches long, it refused to break into smaller pieces for expulsion. We manipulated it to the top of the stomach and made a small incision, revealing what appeared to be a chewed piece of pale-coloured rubber. It appeared that this offending item had blocked the stomach outflow, causing Suzie's bloat.

The foreign body was soon removed and the stomach incision successfully closed. By now Suzie had been under anaesthesia for over two hours and we were increasingly concerned about her condition. And so, without further ado, I began the lengthy process of closing her multi-layered abdominal incisions.

All had proceeded beautifully so far, when the nurse suddenly informed me that Suzie was no longer breathing. "Turn off the anaesthetic gas and check for a heartbeat!" I cried. He was unable to hear the heart beating. Tearing off my bloodied gloves, I grabbed the stethoscope from his hands, and confirmed the deathly silence within Suzie's chest.

We grabbed the 'crash kit' and injected massive doses of adrenaline into Suzie's intravenous drip lines, in a desperate attempt to restart her heart. I manually compressed her chest as quickly as I could, while a nurse manipulated the reservoir bag attached to the anaesthetic machine, providing artificial breaths of pure oxygen every 5-10 seconds. We added a respiratory stimulant to her intravenous lines, but nothing seemed to work, other than a very brief period when her heart gave two slow beats, then stopped again. After 10-15 exhausting minutes we were forced to face the reality that Suzie was not coming back to us.

Mr Jones took the news extremely well. It turned out that the piece of 'rubber' was exactly the size and colour of a 'chew' he had fed Suzie the day before, which had clearly been insufficiently chewed. Mrs Jones, on the other hand, was somewhat hysterical. Suzie had clearly been very much loved, and this elderly couple had no other animals or children living with them.

Breaking news like this is one of the hardest parts of a veterinarian's job. I know that what will haunt me most, however, is the memory of Suzie's eyes, as she gazed at me calmly and trustingly from the X-ray table, her heart rate steadily climbing, matching her increasing discomfort as she went into shock. Suzie never once complained. She was only three, and did not deserve to die.

As the years roll by, I see an ever-increasing stream of old German Shepherds with debilitating arthritis, West Highland White Terriers with painfully inflamed skin allergies, Pugs with breathing difficulties, heat stroke and increased anaesthetic risks, due to their cruelly-shortened faces, Cavalier King Charles Spaniels with progressing heart disease, and other pure-breeds with a wide range of hereditary defects. Now, I am able to add first-hand experience of the life-threatening hazards of giant stomachs, in giant breeds.

Literally hundreds of such anatomical vulnerabilities and deformities exist, associated with virtually every pure breed. The financial and emotional suffering of their human guardians pales in comparison to that experienced by these poor animals, trapped for life in defective bodies, created because someone once thought an unusual dog was aesthetically pleasing, or suited some other human purpose. The cycle is perpetuated whenever an excited new owner pays some thoughtless person to continue breeding such animals. And that is why veterinarians such as I wish people would only realise that the healthiest dogs have always been mixed-breed mutts.

Andrew Knight

Emergency Weight Loss

"Honestly, she gained all that weight just in the last fortnight!" Mrs Smith told me earnestly. I stifled a sigh, which quickly became a grimace as her 60kg dog lowered itself onto my arm once again. Despite numerous, valiant attempts to digitally stimulate her contractions, and two very strong hormonal injections, Sasha showed no signs of voluntarily delivering the puppy I could feel with my fingertips, lodged high up her birth canal. Although its smooth, wet head had passed tantalisingly down my fingers several times, I had been unable to achieve the necessary purchase in the confined and slippery environment, before it retracted frustratingly out of reach.

Meanwhile, Sasha continued to pant, depositing copious volumes of slobber onto my increasingly slippery consult room floor, impeding her foothold and mine. The increasing exhaustion of this gigantic Rottweiler resulted in ever weightier attempts to lower her bulk onto my arm, which were resisted ever more feebly by the increasingly exhausted Mrs Smith and her elderly neighbour, unsuspectingly roused from his bed some hours ago to assist.

It occurred to me that just possibly Mrs Smith might not have been feeding Sasha the healthiest of diets, exercising her regularly, nor have noticed her obesity problem when it had clearly first become evident, at least a year ago. The result was that Sasha's muscles were weak and flabby, and she was quite clearly incapable of giving birth on her own.

This posed a problem, because the efficiency of her circulatory and respiratory systems – which would already be hazardously depressed under anaesthesia – would be further compromised by her excessive fat and poor fitness. This would increase the chances of death for her and her puppies, should we have to conduct the Caesarean section operation, that seemed more and more inevitable as the midnight hours passed.

I was somehow not surprised to learn that Mrs Smith had neither the £1,000+ routinely necessary to pay for such an operation, nor pet insurance to cover the costs of such unexpected medical or surgical requirements. She was, in short, woefully ill equipped to care for Sasha's needs responsibly. However, we were not prepared to let Sasha or her unborn puppies die, which would have been the inevitable natural outcome without surgical intervention. And so, after I had reluctantly placed a call to the head veterinarian at home around midnight, Mrs Smith signed ownership of Sasha over to the practice. We would provide the necessary care, absorbing the costs ourselves, and look after Sasha and her puppies until suitable homes could be found for them.

My exhausted nurse and I quickly prepared Sasha for surgery. We amazed ourselves by somehow managing to manhandle her unconscious bulk on to the operating table, which creaked with protest under the strain. Hastened by my significant concern about Sasha's survival chances, the incision was probably my fastest ever, despite her size, and rapidly exposed the largest uterus I had seen. Massively engorged blood vessels pulsated alarmingly along the length of this gargantuan purple nightmare, which was distended with foetuses and fluid. As I attempted to manoeuvre it into position, the uterus suddenly tore under its own weight, ejecting copious quantities of greenish-black fluid onto the floor, from which it splashed unerringly on to the base of the white designer jeans I had recklessly chosen to wear beneath my surgical gown. *"Thank God I wore my boots!"* I thought, as I cautiously cast a glance at my long-suffering nurse, intently monitoring the anaesthetic. She would be here until 6 am scrubbing the walls.

At least the foetuses were easier to remove. Eight voluminous placental splashes later, accompanied by much frantic rubbing by the nurse (to simulate the mother's licking), and the addition of a few drops of respiratory stimulant under little puppy tongues, five tiny, wet and apparently very hungry Rottweiler puppies squeaked vigorously at the world. Three had not survived, victims of the prolonged, unsuccessful labour prior to the op.

Thankfully, Sasha had also survived, and, with the elimination of her uterus – as well as copious quantities of fat enthusiastically removed during my incision – had lost an impressive 5 kg! I considered it the start of her emergency weight loss programme. She had made a good beginning.

Unfortunately, however, it was not to be enough, because Sasha accidentally suffocated a puppy a night, for the next two nights, under her excessive weight. Although common in modern sows, which are intentionally bred for their bulk, I had never encountered this problem before in a dog! After a certain amount of head-scratching, we soon arrived at a logical solution. If Sasha was built like a sow, we would treat her like one! Accordingly, we used wooden planks to build crawl spaces around her, under which her three surviving puppies were able to escape crushing and suffocation when she rolled. It must have worked, because all remaining puppies survived. Her nursing and veterinary staff also narrowly survived, albeit in a rather dishevelled state, thanks to copious quantities of coffee and dark chocolate, mixed with a pitifully small amount of sleep.

It was, therefore, with a certain amount of satisfaction that I noted Mrs Smith's profoundly shaken tone, when I placed a courtesy call to inform her that Sasha had survived her operation. The traumatic, late-night ordeal had clearly instilled in her a much sounder understanding of the magnitude of the commitment involved in caring for – let alone breeding – a dog. Considerable time, effort and financial resources, not to mention suitable housing, are required to responsibly care for an animal companion. In both effort and reward, the commitment is somewhat similar to raising a child, and should remain for the animal's lifetime.

In this case Mrs Smith had lost her beloved companion, and by overfeeding and under-exercising Sasha – probably through misguided kindness – had needlessly endangered her life, as well as the lives of her puppies, the majority of which had not survived. Thankfully, she had no intention of acquiring another dog any time soon.

Saving individual animal lives is perhaps the most rewarding part of a veterinarian's job. Cases like Sasha's demonstrate, however, that perhaps the most important part is the education of animal guardians about the basics of responsible pet care, namely: diet and exercise, vaccinations and annual checkups, external and internal parasite control, dental care, neutering, socialisation and behavioural training, adequate space and environmental enrichment, the provision of company for social species, the specialised needs of exotic species, and the wisdom of pet insurance.

We can save the most lives using the least resources, by educating guardians about such preventative healthcare measures, which demonstrates the importance of a fact well-known to veterinary educators, but little-known outside the profession: communication and interpersonal skills are even more vital to practising veterinarians, than surgical or other technical skills. The former are frequently challenged to the utmost, within routine veterinary practice.

Andrew Knight

Hetty

As many of you may be aware – a lot of West Highland White Terriers suffer from skin disease. Little Hetty had an awful problem with her skin and also a food sensitivity. From a young age she had visited the practice with itchy skin and severe hair loss, which became greasier, thickened and darkened over time. Normal skin should be pink and healthy in appearance, but diseased skin becomes darker as pigment is deposited due to the inflammatory process.

The most common cause of the problem in Westies is an allergy of some sort, often to inhaled allergens. All too many Westies come in to see us suffering from such bad skin and it is recognised that the problem may be inherited, that is, the tendency to develop this problem can be passed on genetically between the bitch (or dog) and the pups. Sadly, after lengthy investigations (skin scrapings, parasite testing and control, diet trials and referral to a specialist) many of them end up on steroids to suppress the itch. Long-term steroid treatment can cause many problems for the dog, and can lead to a condition called Cushing's Disease.

However time and time again one finds oneself handing out steroids and antibiotics to try and control a raging skin condition in these lovely little dogs. Some owners cannot bear to see the dog scratching and scratching over and over again, and are very happy for us to do everything we can to investigate the problem. However, other owners seem oblivious to their pet's suffering and refuse my treatment recommendations with a flippant "well lots of Westies look like this – it's the breed". This often occurs when I suggest referring an animal to see a specialist because skin investigations in particular, can be lengthy and costly.

Hetty too, had worked her way down the diagnostic protocol list for her itchy skin and also her intermittent diarrhoea and sickness. Fortunately, we discovered that a novel prescription diet made by a company specialising in prescription foods for various different conditions worked well for her. The ingredients of this diet are different to those in 'off the shelf' dog foods, the idea being that if the dog has not been exposed to the ingredients before, it won't react to cause sensitive bowels or itchy skin. Hetty's itching and diarrhoea stopped altogether and in time her hair slowly grew back. You would never have known that she had been so bald in the past!

However with Hetty being of such a nice nature, her owner decided it would be nice to have a litter of puppies from her. Unfortunately she did not seek our advice first before mating Hetty. So many Westies have bad skin; it is wise to only breed from animals that do not suffer from this problem. The owner did not consider that Hetty's pups might also suffer from such severe skin disease; she wasn't aware of the morals behind responsible breeding and had only considered the little dog's good temperament in her decision to breed.

The first we knew about Hetty being pregnant was when the owner rang to ask us if there was anything extra or any supplements she needed to feed her through the pregnancy. Unfortunately for Hetty, her prescription dog food keeping her in such good-looking condition was too low in protein to support pregnancy. Despite a lengthy discussion with the producers of the diet and their veterinary support team they recommended that the diet was not fed to the dog. We informed the client of this who had to make a choice – feed the diet and risk losing the puppies, or stop feeding the diet in which case Hetty would revert to her previous state of itching and diarrhoea.

The owner desperately wanted the puppies so she decided to stop feeding the diet and give her one more suitable for the pregnancy. As Hetty neared her due date the vomiting and diarrhoea became progressively worse and her hair began to once again become patchy.

Despite her illness, Hetty carried her pups to term. When she was whelping (the term used to describe the birthing process in dogs), the owner became concerned about her lack of progress because she delivered the first two pups uneventfully, but did not seem to be progressing thereafter. So she came down to the surgery for observation and any necessary intervention.

When she passed the third pup, in her keenness to mother the new arrival, Hetty chewed too far along the naval cord. I heard a shout from the owner in the surgery room where Hetty had been enjoying time by the radiator with a blanket whilst she gave birth. The puppy's guts had herniated.

As quickly as we could, I anaesthetised the puppy using a facemask and anaesthetic gas. It is a risky procedure anaesthetising a newborn pup because they metabolise anaesthetic very quickly and they can wake up in an instant, but if they are given too much anaesthetic, it may kill them.

The surgery to replace the intestines and stitch up the hole in her umbilicus (belly button) was very difficult, mainly due to the size of the puppy and the anaesthetic difficulty, but thankfully the tiny pup survived and eventually made a nice pet. Not many puppies are so lucky; if this had happened at the client's home the pup would likely not even have survived the journey to the surgery. Hetty's owner was very grateful and took Hetty home with five live puppies.

All the puppies were sold except for one. As chance would have it, the only puppy that developed a skin condition was the one she kept. At just three weeks of age, it came in scratching. Treatment for such a young puppy was limited and the condition progressed. The puppy grew older and despite thorough investigations and treatments, and eating the same special diet as Hetty its skin remained out of control.

There was not any more that we could do so we offered referral to see a skin specialist, which the owner declined to our dismay.

Having been through so much with Hetty (and after we had repeatedly explained to the owner how the condition could be passed on genetically) I was disappointed when the owner said to my colleague in a consultation for the scratching pup, who was now one year old, "Oh I know I shouldn't but it would be nice to use him as a stud dog just once – he's just got such a lovely character."

I was shocked that the owner would even consider this, given her experiences with both Hetty and her pup suffering so severely from skin disease. Aside from the animals' suffering, she had almost lost Hetty during pregnancy. The costs involved to manage conditions such as this are great and she would have to deal with the dishonesty of selling someone else a problem puppy. Yet she still wanted to use the dog as a stud dog – just once.

We tried our best to convince her against breeding with the male pup. At first we thought we had lost the battle but eventually we were able to breath a sigh of relief when she phoned a week later to book the dog in for his castration.

This time, our advice was heeded and the message got through to the owner, but we are not always so successful in helping owners to make the correct, responsible decisions. People will listen to our advice, but they often choose not to follow it and I have had to learn to accept this in order to cope with the job. At the end of the day, 'we can take a horse to water, but we can't make it drink' as the saying goes!

As an interesting aside, Hetty's mum, a keen baker, has struck an interesting bargain with my boss! She does not pay for her prescription dog food, but rather she bakes his own personal prescription diet of gluten free cakes each week as he has a gluten allergy. We think this is a perfect trade-off and means there is cake for everyone at coffee time!

Anonymous

The English Patients

At long last I opened my own practice and the highlights included pinning a heron's broken wing, murine plastic surgery (stitching up the face of a mouse rescued from the cat), a Caesarean on a marmoset and mending a dog's tibial fracture using a graft of chips made from the animal's tail end vertebrae.

Let me tell you about this last mentioned most interesting case ...

A dog was brought into the surgery that had been treated elsewhere for a broken leg but the fracture refused to heal properly. Instead of knitting together with solid bone, soft cartilage had been formed, with the result that every time the dog put weight on the limb the bone was distorted.

The presence of cartilage at the fracture site, coupled with the absence of pain and continued weight bearing, prevented proper healing. I decided to take away all the unhealthy tissue (about 2cm) but in order to avoid shortening of the leg the gap was packed tightly with crushed bone. This was made from an excised rib and from vertebrae, obtained by amputating the dog's tail.

The bone ends were also kept in place by using a metal plate screwed to the outside of the bone and a pin passed down the marrow cavity.

The operation worked well and when the pin was removed three months later healing was complete.

Cutting bits off animal's tails for appearance sake has always seemed the height of barbarity to me, especially in countries where sentimentality about pets is sometimes taken to extremes. The fact that the tails of undocked dogs could be useful for future grafting procedures is an added reason against the procedure.

Another case too was destined to give me a great deal of pleasure. One day a small mongrel dog, half black Labrador, was brought into the surgery with a broken femur. These fractures are usually easy to repair but for some reason this one just would not heal. I tried everything, first a pin down the marrow cavity, then a plate screwed to the bone and finally a double plate, one on each side of the bone with bolts going between the two plates. But one setback followed another and eventually I just had to admit defeat.

With a heavy heart I discussed the matter with the owners and it was decided to amputate the limb. This however is not a major catastrophe in dogs because they cope remarkably well on three legs, especially if the missing one is a hind leg. After all, a dog with three legs still has one more than we have!

I am not soppy about dogs but there was something about this dog's spirit that I could not help admiring. His tail wagged incessantly and he seemed to overflow with enjoyment. His eyes were as shiny as I have ever seen, and he looked directly at people as if he was doing everything he could to please.

Once he'd had his leg taken off I took him home and kept him in my bedroom overnight. He whimpered softly now and then and I spent several hours kneeling beside him, holding his body against mine, feeling guilty and trying to take some of the pain. In years to come something of a bond grew between us and I would like to think he remembered that night as I did.

The dog made a good recovery but imagine my disappointment when the owners said they could not face the sight of a three-legged dog and wanted him put to sleep. I just could not do it, so I said I would keep him myself.

He had previously been named 'Lupo' (dog) but I misheard this and thought his name was 'Loophole'. The new name stuck and Loophole turned out a most wonderfully game, communicative and happy dog.

He spent some of his time in the company of a large and strong golden Labrador but was so well adjusted to his disability that he was even more agile than his companion. He ran almost without a limp and on casual glance you could quite easily miss the fact that he had only three legs.

Much as Loophole loved people he loved the fairer sex of his own species more. If there were a bitch on heat anywhere in a radius of 10 miles, Loophole would be gone for days on end to camp outside his heartthrob's door and pounce on her if she managed to escape the vigilance of her owners.

Eventually there would come a telephone call from an irate dog owner asking us to please collect our dog and I had to go along, full of apologies, to drag our recalcitrant lover-dog home.

Sometimes Loophole would be successful and on such occasions would return at daybreak after his night on the tiles. There would be a sound outside our back door, half a bark, half tired whimper, and when I opened it Loophole would run straight past me, and looking neither to the left or right make straight for his basket, curl up and go sound asleep.

We are warned (for some reason) to avoid interpreting animal behaviour as we would a person's but nonetheless every bachelor will recognise that wonderful feeling of exhausted happiness that suffuses your every fibre as you drop off to sleep after a successful conquest.

We moved away from the area shortly afterwards, which was fortunate because if there were a spate of three-legged puppies born I could scarcely have denied Loophole's responsibility. After we moved, we did of course castrate him but he still wanders off occasionally. At least now he won't be able to father any unwanted puppies.

Leonard Black

The Dog Fight

A call came into the surgery from a rather distraught lady – Mrs Thomas. The two dogs she was looking after for her daughter, whilst she was away, were fighting and she could not stop them. All she had managed to do was put the dogs outside and in a panicked state she had also phoned the police.

I was able to set off straight away and I took with me our practice nurse Hannah, who was quite keen to come for the adventure, as it seemed like it was going to be an interesting visit. We took the dogcatcher (a pole with an adjustable loop on the end), a selection of muzzles and some antibiotic tablets. My car already contained an 'examination kit' and a 'Caesar kit' and, whilst these were aimed at farm animal practice, I could use them to treat the dogs if needed. Anything major and I would have to transport the dogs back to the surgery for treatment.

An elderly lady, who must have been in her eighties, met us at the door of an isolated detached house in the countryside. She looked somewhat shocked but welcomed us into the house. Hannah followed me in carrying the dogcatcher and muzzles. As I understood it, the police had also been called but I had beaten them to it and there was no sign of them yet. There were spots of blood all the way through the house from the door to the back yard where the dogs were now shut. I peered through the window at the dogs, who were now standing still, looking back at me, all fighting finished with.

Mrs Thomas explained that she had been looking after the dogs for her daughter who was away for another two weeks in Turkey. The dogs were two Dobermans – brother and sister – who were known to fight at times, so the daughter had left Mrs Thomas two muzzles to put on the dogs should they start to misbehave. Apparently the two dogs had started to growl at each other and then it had got out of hand and they had started biting at each other. Mrs Thomas had been unable to get the muzzles on the dogs when the growling started and once they started biting, she had been unable to do anything except push the dogs outside the house and into the back yard. Being such an old lady, she had not had the strength to separate the two big dogs.

"I couldn't stop them, they knocked me against the kitchen worktop."

I asked if the dogs were all right with people – I didn't want to get savaged the minute I set foot into the yard. It turned out that neither dog had ever bitten a person before so I entered the yard. To my surprise my keen assistant was not so keen to follow me in, despite having charge of the dogcatcher. Instead she shut the door after me and peered through the window with her face surrounded by the loop of the dog catcher. 'Great,' I thought, 'don't look out for me will you!'

Both the dogs were quiet and they let me get close enough to examine them even with no one holding them. One had a few cuts on its neck and legs, nothing major and the other had a cut on its ear. As both dogs seemed fine, I decided that they would be OK on antibiotic cover, nothing else would be needed. I returned to Hannah and Mrs Thomas, who had been watching me through the kitchen window.

Hannah was already talking to Mrs Thomas. "Are you sure you're going to be all right looking after them for another two weeks?"

Mrs Thomas was insistent that she would be OK, but we both noticed that she seemed to be nursing her hand. It looked swollen and was already starting to bruise.

"You should get that hand seen to at the doctor's." I said.

"Oh, no I'll be all right, thank you."

"You don't look OK" said Hannah, "are you going to go to the doctor's?"

"I don't have a car," replied Mrs Thomas. We offered to drive Mrs Thomas to the doctor's but she refused. I felt we had pushed her enough as she looked like she was about to cry. We left Mrs Thomas with some tablets for the two dogs and on the walk out to the car we discussed how she should have gone to the doctor's.

Just as we were getting in the car, a police car arrived. We went to speak to the policeman and explained that the dogs had stopped fighting and were OK although Mrs Thomas had hurt her hand.

He wanted to see Mrs Thomas anyway as I had told him about her hand, so we all went back to the house. The policeman spoke to Mrs Thomas and asked if she was all right and how was her hand. Mrs Thomas again said she was fine although there were tears welling up in her eyes.

"How are you going to look after the dogs," he asked. We could all see that Mrs Thomas was not going to give in despite our best efforts to look after her. Elderly people can be quite stubborn at times and I felt we were all starting to bully her. After a pause we left at the initiation of the policeman. Outside he discussed with us – "It's a big place for such an elderly lady to look after, she obviously can't drive so she can't get anywhere. I think it was very unfair of her daughter to expect her to look after those two big dogs for a month. I could take the dogs and have them put in kennels." I wasn't really sure if he wanted my input on this – whether it was a sort of question. He seemed to be debating whether he should remove the dogs or not. I couldn't really help, as I had no such powers or knew any laws regarding this – it was his responsibility.

He decided in the end to leave the dogs with Mrs Thomas and we parted to go our separate ways. I guess, being an elderly lady Mrs Thomas wanted to fight against her age and did not want to feel that she had lost her independence or capabilities. It looked like she was refusing to give up and also did not want her daughter to know she had struggled with the dogs.

Anonymous

Chapter 4 – Emotional Stories

A Shocking Truth

Mars was a mixed breed terrier type dog belonging to a middle-aged couple called Mr and Mrs Carson. They had been particularly impressed with a consult in which I had seen their dog. Mars needed to lose some weight and Mr and Mrs Carson were keen on home-made diets. I had gone to the effort of researching some home-made obesity diets and had sent them a few written copies by post. At the time I couldn't find anything wrong with Mars apart from his increasing weight, for which I hoped the new diets and a little more exercise would help.

However Mars was still gaining weight and came back into the surgery a month later, but now his coat was starting to go patchy with some of his hair starting to fall out. By now he was also off his food and vomiting what little he had tried to eat. My colleague started a consult but I was happy to take over the case when Mars was admitted for a blood sample and an X-ray to try and get to the bottom of the problem, as it had been going on for some time now. Having seen Mars before in our other surgery branch I was keen to find out what his ailment was.

We checked Mars over and sedated him for the X-ray, not only to keep him still on the X-ray plate but also because he was quite aggressive so it would make taking a blood sample easier and less stressful. Apart from the weight gain and strange hair there was nothing else to note on physical examination. We went ahead and took an X-ray and a blood sample.

We injected Mars on the operating room table to reverse the sedative we had given earlier and after a couple of minutes he started to wake up, lifting his head. The practice nurse had been helping me with the bloods and she was supervising Mars on the table as he came round and I was chatting to her as I was waiting. No sooner had he lifted his head, a dreadful event occurred and in a split second Mars had died in our arms. I couldn't believe it, it happened so fast. He must have died of an extremely acute internal incident such as a heart attack. I was shocked – he had been fine all throughout his sedation and we had finished, he had been reversed and was starting to wake up. I was devastated, we sedate dogs all the time and this happens to only a very small percentage of animals undergoing any form of anaesthetic. The owners had left the dog in my care and were expecting him home in a few hours.

I rang them straight away as I often find that dealing with a difficult or upsetting situation at the time closes an event for you and gives the client a genuine response not a prepared speech.

I dialled the number and reported the shocking event. Mrs Carson burst into tears and had no response, after a minute she put her husband on. The news had shocked her as much as if it had been her child. As she had been unable to say anything at all, I had to repeat the news to her husband. He too cried but was still able to speak and I managed to explain as best I could what had happened.

I had lunch hour to recover before Mr Carson picked up Mars later on that day to bury his pet at home. He made pleasantries when he arrived and as I carried the dog out to the car he asked, "How is the Mondeo going? That's yours over there isn't it?" He thanked me and got in his car. "I know you did your best."

I think his car comment was a way of coping at the time but it did surprise me that he could identify the car as mine especially as I had not previously done a house call; he had no reason to know that.

I appreciated him thanking me for my best efforts though I still felt upset about what had happened to Mars.

Unfortunately it was one of those things – there is a risk with every sedative and anaesthetic. And whilst most dogs are fine, once in a while an animal dies as a result and for an unknown reason even if it is just a routine castrate. The effect is shocking for both the vet and the client. This must be one of the most upsetting things that can happen to a vet, and then to have to report the unexpected death to the owner. Most clients are aware of anaesthetic risks in relation to an older animal but many forget the risk, albeit small, for a younger animal or a routine neuter operation. That is why we always ask our clients to sign a consent form stating that there is always a risk associated with any anaesthetic, which should never be taken for granted.

Anonymous

I Do Understand – I Really Do

Zack was beautiful, a three month old seal point Siamese kitten with bright blue eyes. And so very friendly – he would purr and roll around on my consulting table whenever his owner brought him in. Mrs Morris herself was not so easy to get on with. She could be quite abrupt and was always very measured and guarded when she spoke to me. She never seemed to trust anyone at the practice completely and expected the worst from people. She always seemed to be unhappy, although her eyes would light up whenever she looked at Zack. I clearly saw Mrs Morris' lack of enthusiasm for life and thought that this may be why she seemed quite rude on occasion. Zack seemed to be one of her few sources of joy in the world.

When Zack became unwell, Mrs Morris became demanding and impatient during the consultation with me. I could see how afraid she was of losing him. I had to admit Zack for further testing and emergency supportive treatments, because his condition had come on so rapidly. Sadly, despite our very best efforts, we had to put Zack to sleep because he was suffering from severe anaemia secondary to Feline Leukaemia. I arranged an appointment so that Mrs Morris could come and be with Zack as we put him to sleep. He went very peacefully in her arms, it was so very sad to see and yet at least poor Zack wasn't suffering any more. Mrs Morris had an empty, hopeless look in her eyes. She couldn't quite believe it and she shook her head faintly from side to side the whole time as she cradled him in her arms.

I put my hand on hers, "I am so sorry, I understand how hard it is," I said with genuine sympathy.

She looked angry and rounded on me, "No you don't, how can you? You don't understand. He's helped me ... he ... helped ... me ..." tears welled in her eyes as she glared at me.

But I was used to dealing with grief – that of other people and my own. Like many others at such times, Mrs Morris' anger at losing Zack had to be directed somewhere. I knew then that Mrs Morris was suffering from depression, just as I had done not so long ago.

"I do understand, I really do," I said, nodding and looking at her. I put my arm around her. She grabbed me back in a hug and cried for some time on my shoulder. I had a busy surgery waiting outside, but Mrs Morris needed my time. My boss wouldn't agree with me, I am sure. He would say that it's not our job to comfort people. But sometimes compassion takes priority over business issues in my opinion.

After a few minutes she stopped crying and said, "I'll never have another one."

I smiled, understanding her, "I know it seems unbearable just now, but it does get easier. In time, you must get yourself another kitten. You've been so very unlucky this time."

She kept shaking her head at the thought of 'replacing' Zack, but I knew it was really important to plant that seed straight away. Often, people will cut themselves off from the joy of owning an animal because they find the grief of losing them so difficult. We can never replace our little friends, but we can form new bonds, and give an animal a much needed loving home. When Mrs Morris was ready, I let her leave in privacy through the back door rather than walking through our busy waiting room. As she left, I squeezed her hand and said, "You will be OK." She looked back with a reticent smile and nodded lightly. I made sure she had someone waiting in the car to give her a lift and then went to my computer to type up my notes – "Anaemia, Feline Leukaemia positive. Prognosis dire. Euthanasia on welfare grounds" was all I needed to type.

I cleaned my consulting room and gently took Zack to the back room prep area where I got him ready for his cremation. I took a deep breath and mentally shook myself before going out into the waiting room to continue with my consults,

"Mrs Robinson with Bella please."

I smiled as the young Lurcher bounded up to me – looking like Bambi in the film when he first learned to walk.

"I'm sorry to keep you waiting. Now what can we do for you today?"

About three weeks later, I felt delighted when I saw 'Toby Morris – Kitten – 1st vaccination' on my computer screen during my morning appointments. When Mrs Morris came in she was smiling – she looked better than I had ever seen her before. As she opened the box, she brimmed with pride over her new addition. Toby was (and still is) a beautiful cream Siamese. We agreed to test him for Feline Leukaemia virus before we did anything else – the result came back all clear – and then we started his vaccination course.

Mrs Morris started to thank me for being kind to her the other week, but I stopped her. Seeing her so happy with Toby was all the thanks I needed. Of course, I couldn't guarantee Toby's health in the future. But, like everything else in life, we have to keep 'getting back on our bike' and not give up because something bad has happened to us. I felt grateful that I could use my own negative experiences to help another person – it's a real gift for me to have the honour of doing so.

Mhairi Cameron

Old Ethel

It had been a quiet evening on call, but first thing on Tuesday morning the phone rang. I had to go out on a visit to see an elderly lady living way out 'in the sticks'. Although I phoned her before I set off, I could not figure out what the problem might be. All she kept saying was that her dog was ill and it needed a 'tonic'. I was not quite sure what she meant by a tonic, but I agreed to set off immediately as she sounded very concerned about her dog. Although it was 8.00am by the time I left, the owner said it would be impossible for her to get to the surgery when it opened at 9.00am just an hour later. I knew I would miss the first morning consults of the day but my colleagues would be at the surgery and could start without me.

Fortunately I was familiar with the area and the owner had given me good directions, so I found the house quite easily. She was a very pleasant elderly lady who lived on her own and she was pleased to see me. I followed her through the house to the kitchen where there was a small Jack Russell Terrier lying in a comfortable wicker basket lined with blankets beside an 'aga' (an old style oven which also provides heating for the house).

I took a history from the lady, which was fairly brief as she was not able to tell me much except that her dog, Jody, was very quiet, just lying in her basket most of the day and only getting up to drink. Jody was a 12-year-old entire bitch, which means that she had not been neutered.

The poor little dog was very dehydrated, her skin remaining tented when I pinched it. She was pale and had a slight temperature and she boarded her abdomen (tensed up her muscles) when I tried to feel her tummy, making it difficult to feel anything that could help me identify her problem. I realised that one of the main possible causes of Jody's illness was a condition called 'pyometra' (an infection of the uterus which causes it to fill with pus). This problem tends to occur in older animals and it typically happens in the weeks after the bitch's season.

With further questioning I discovered that Jody had, in fact, been in season a few weeks earlier. I explained to her owner that I would need to do some further tests, such as an ultrasound scan or X-ray, and a blood sample, to confirm my suspicions, and that Jody was seriously unwell and needed further treatment immediately. If, indeed, it were a pyometra we would then have to do emergency surgery to remove the uterus.

Although I explained as best I could, I don't think Jody's owner fully understood. She was very elderly, moved around with some difficulty and was a little hard of hearing. She asked me again if I could give the dog a tonic to make her better. I replied that whilst antibiotics may help a little, in the very short term, Jody was really very sick and we would have to do a full 'workup' to confirm the problem, which could be quite costly. Our only options were either immediate treatment or that we must put Jody to sleep to prevent her from suffering further.

The old lady, whose name I discovered was Ethel, was upset by my suggestion of putting Jody to sleep and I could see tears forming in her eyes. There was silence for a minute before she spoke, her voice now trembling. She explained that she had recently lost her husband and that her son had also passed on, she did have other animals previously too, which she seemed to consider as her only family, but she had also lost them slowly over the past few months.

"Jody is all I've got left," she sobbed.

I felt terrible upsetting Ethel by suggesting that I euthanase her last companion. But I also realised how sick Jody was, and there was a real risk I might run up an expensive bill for an old pensioner only to have the same, tragic outcome in the end. I feared that Jody was so ill that she might not survive any treatment. It really had to be her decision and I spent considerable time repeating again what the options were and discussing them in full with her.

Ethel pleaded with me to do what I could for her dog. So I agreed to take Jody back to the surgery in my car for further investigation and treatment. As I left the house, I could see in my interior mirror, Ethel peering out through the kitchen window with a handkerchief in her hand, waving goodbye to Jody. I spent the whole drive back wondering whether I had done the right thing in agreeing to try for Jody, but I didn't feel I had any other option.

Jody was so badly dehydrated it was not possible to gain access to the vein in her small leg. We eventually had to put nearly a whole bag of fluids under her skin, which would rehydrate her much more slowly, but this worked and an hour later, we succeeded in catheterising her vein.

To my surprise, our office staff were not very supportive of my attempts to help Jody – rather they were more concerned about the bill when I told them how sick she was and it was likely to be a pyometra. They thought I should just have put Jody to sleep. Having been at the practice a lot longer than I had, I guess they had seen many last desperate attempts with an unsuccessful outcome. But they had no idea how much Jody meant to Ethel.

I ultrasound scanned Jody's abdomen to confirm my suspected diagnosis of pyometra, as this was the most cost effective test to perform. Again the office staff tried to persuade me to put her down! I rang the old lady, feeling very pressured by the office staff not to undertake the surgery that Jody so desperately needed. She picked up the phone quickly and broke down into tears. She was insistent on me trying to do my best for her little companion. Altogether I must have rung her at least three times before the operation. trying to coax her to put Jody to sleep. But Ethel simply wouldn't consent to me putting Jody to sleep, so my only option was to proceed with surgery.

I operated that morning to remove her uterus, which was grossly enlarged from the pus inside it. I operated with just one other member of staff in the room – the rest remained disapprovingly at the front in reception. Hannah was more sympathetic and offered to help. I prayed throughout the whole operation that the little terrier would make it for old Ethel's sake.

Jody came round fine from the general anaesthetic, which was a relief. When I rang Ethel to say that she had pulled through the operation, she cried with joy at the news. I told her that Jody was not out of the woods yet and still had to make it through the next few days.

I am delighted to report that Jody made a good recovery and I had the pleasure of removing her stitches ten days later. However the bill came to several hundred pounds, even though I knocked off the out of hours visit that I had done before opening hours. Despite Jody's recovery and Ethel being so delighted, the office staff still made it clear that they disapproved of me running up a large bill for a pensioner and I found this difficult to deal with. They had not met or even spoken to Ethel on the phone. They had not heard how desperate she was to keep Jody that bit longer, especially after recently losing her husband. They had no empathy at all with the client. I do the best I can for both the animal and the owner, and in this case I felt for Ethel and I too had wanted Jody to survive.

I had discounted the bill as much as I could by calling the out of hours time as my own time. I don't know how much longer Jody lived for as I have not seen or heard from Ethel since the day I took the stitches out, but I still wonder whether I did the right thing. It would have taken her many months to pay her bill when her only income was her pension.

We often have to deal with elderly owners, and in many cases, they are incredibly lonely and the pet is all they have got. It can be very hard to deal with this situation and often the pet is also very old. I often wish that we had a practice policy that allowed our elderly pensioners to receive a discount. At the moment there is nothing in place for this at our surgery; although we do occasionally knock some money off when the boss's back is turned, such as I did with waiving the out of hours visit!

Anonymous

All's Well that Ends Well

It was as bleak a December day as you could imagine. The sky was heavy with dark cloud. The rain drummed incessantly on the surgery window panes and the raw, icy wind blew straight down from the Siberian steppes.

As is so often the case, the bad weather kept most of the clients at home and there was only one person in the waiting room: a little old lady, emaciated and slightly bent, but with a pleasant, bright face. On invitation, she came into the consulting room dragging a small, wet and reluctant pooch.

The dog had only a minor ailment that was quickly attended to. The woman then said that the time was fast approaching when she would have to have the dog put to sleep and could I please tell her what the procedure would entail. As things were quiet I had plenty of time and I was pleased to set her mind at ease about a topic which most animal lovers view with apprehension. So in some detail I described just what would happen, from the start of the fatal day when she could give tranquillisers to the dog with a good breakfast, through to the kindest of all injections and then to the time three weeks later when she could, if she wished, have the ashes back in a small box to place on the mantle shelf or bury in the garden.

Both she and the dog listened attentively and then, as is often so, she said what a pity it was that a similar kind and gentle end was not available for people. When I said I agreed wholeheartedly it seemed to open a floodgate and she embarked on a most sad diatribe about all her relatives and friends who had died in terrible circumstances. The poor woman had had a string of awful experiences. First one relative and then another had suffered appalling, prolonged and agonising deaths about which she spared me no detail. It went on and on and as soon as one relative was safely laid to rest the next started to develop the dreaded symptoms that were to end in the same way.

Eventually she was almost in tears and to tell the truth, so was I; but enough was enough and I managed to steer her toward the door. With one hand on the doorknob she suddenly turned, her eyes brightening with something remembered. I waited, my heart sinking a little further.

"Oh yes," she said, "and a very merry Christmas to you" as she opened the door and walked quickly out.

Leonard Black

There was Nothing I Could Do to Help

As I was finishing my last phone call of the day with a client, Michelle was just starting to lock all the doors when in walked a woman with a German Shepherd dog slowly following her. Distracted from what I was saying on the phone I got a general gist of what was being said. Just as I had thought – she was asking if there was a vet still here and could she be seen.

Disgruntled that I thought I'd done my last consult and was just ringing a client to report some blood results before leaving for home, I hung up the phone. Yet another one had walked in without an appointment right on closing time expecting to be seen.

I looked grumpily at the woman only to see that her face looked sad and her eyes were watery although there were no tears. The dog was lying at her feet and it's demeanour looked awful. I immediately changed my expression as the woman looked upset and apologised for just turning up.

We went into the consult room and I watched the dog walk in behind us. It was extremely thin and was so weak that it crouched and staggered as it walked. The dog looked old, weak and sick. I took a history. The client explained that the dog had anal furunculosis – a nasty painful condition whereby fistulas (holes) form around the dog's anus, that can be managed to an extent with drugs but cannot be cured. Treatment for this condition is also very expensive. The dog had nearly run out of tablets and the client wanted some more. She also wanted to know why the dog was not eating and was so thin and whether the anal furunculosis was also causing the loss of weight.

I quickly lifted the dog's tail and sure enough there were 'holes' around its anus, which were moist, red and very angry. I then examined the rest of the dog. She was so thin that it was possible to feel every bone. Her muscles had wasted away which was why she was so weak she could hardly stand. When it came to feeling her abdomen I discovered a large, solid mass. In such a thin dog it must have been filling most of her abdomen. This was almost certainly going to be a tumour, and was most likely causing the loss of appetite and weight.

I explained to the client that the dog was extremely ill and I got her to feel the large mass in her abdomen. I explained that even with exploratory surgery she was so ill she would be unlikely to survive an operation to examine her guts and even then it might not be possible to remove the mass. I also explained that the dog had metabolised her own body fat and now most of her muscle mass too. She was so starved of food that effectively she was using her own body to "feed the tumour" growing inside her and she was quickly wasting away to nothing.

The dog was in such a pitiful state. It was all that she could do to just lie there on the floor – she didn't care about any of her surroundings or respond to anyone. The best thing for the poor dog was to put her out of her misery and euthanase her.

Then came the clanger – the client turned out to be looking after the dog and was not the owner. Worse still several people looked after the dog. The actual owner had been in some trouble and according to our computer notes from a previous consult for the dog's anal furunculosis, was in jail! I explained to the client that the dog really should be put down and I would not expect her to survive much longer than a couple of days in the sorry state she was in.

Unfortunately the client replied that she could not give permission for the dog to be put down and would not be able to sign a consent form. I asked her if she could contact the owner. She replied with tears running down her face, "I can contact them but I don't know when I will be able to get hold of them. It might take a week, she's not going to last that long is she?"

I had obviously managed to get through to the client just how bad the dog actually was, although I suspect she knew from the minute she walked in what I was going to recommend.

For the time being, whilst she made efforts to contact the owner, the best I could do was blast the dog with quite a high dose of long-acting steroids to act as a painkiller and an immunosupressant. I also gave the client a few tins of liquid dog food to try and syringe down its throat and asked her to please give us a call when she had obtained permission to euthanase the dog.

The woman paid for the consult and left. I turned to look at Michelle who was sat at the desk waiting to go home, "Don't say anything, I can't bear the thought." I could see how upset Michelle was over how the dog looked. "I would have put it down if I had been looking after the dog." Michelle keeps her own dogs and being a single woman is very passionate about the care that dogs should receive. Her dogs are all she talks about.

I don't know exactly how the woman's story all fits together as to why different people were looking after the dog, and why it was always her who brought the dog to the vets and paid for the treatment – although she did say the owners couldn't afford the expensive tablets all the time. I didn't know why, when she was caring for the dog she did not have permission to euthanase it. Parts of the story did not add up but there was no way I could confiscate the dog or euthanase it without permission.

As a vet it was disappointing not to be able to do the right thing for the dog. It felt like I had failed, Michelle was upset, the client showed some degree of upset and I felt there was nothing else I could do at present. It felt like the client had come in wanting me to put her down, like I could somehow take the dog off her. She was obviously afraid of giving permission or had been told specifically not to have the dog euthanased. I rang a vet helpline that night for advice on the legal aspects of whether it was possible to euthanase a dog without consent of the owner.

The client bringing the dog in specifically indicated that she could not give consent. Whilst some vets may have considered calling the RSPCA, I felt that this would be inappropriate given the unusual circumstances and I feel that the carer of the dog was doing their best under difficult circumstances. The dog was ill but not neglected. Whilst the dog was very skinny I know how quickly a dog with such a large tumour can lose condition for I have seen the rapid deterioration myself in another case.

It must also be respected that not all people believe in euthanasia and for some there is a great difficulty in letting go. Some even need time to come to terms with the idea first and will call us again later as I hoped would be the case with this dog.

I gave a professional opinion that evening, but ultimately it was the client's responsibility for contacting the owner or allowing our practice to do so as soon as possible.

Many people say that it must be the hardest part of our job to euthanase an animal. However most people I feel are wrong with this assumption. Most of the time you are safe in the knowledge that you are doing the right thing and preventing the animal from suffering. Very rarely are you asked to put down a healthy pet. Occasionally it may be a vicious dog that has bitten a family member. Dogs like this have no place in society when they have the potential to injure a child. There are plenty of other pleasant dogs to be kept. The process of euthanasia is kind as it is an overdose of anaesthetic and the animal falls asleep and doesn't wake up. What can be harder to deal with are the emotions of clients if they remain present at the time. Sometimes you can empathise with them so much you can feel a lump in your own throat, after all most people know what it is like to have lost a beloved pet. It is recognised now that the loss of a pet can cause such distress and there are help lines that owners can call to help them get over the bereavement.

Anonymous

Chapter 5 - Vets' Travelling Days

Momo

The year 2007 had a bad start for me. In the space of three short weeks in January, I had split up from my fiancé, sold my half of our house and rehomed my beautiful Lurcher, Loocy, because the new house I was to lodge in was not suitable for dogs. The whole experience knocked me for six.

I decided to go to Nepal on a whim really, but it turned out to be one of my better impulse decisions!

I spent three weeks in Kathmandu neutering and treating the street dogs of the country's capital. Without any form of population control, the stray dog population would continue to expand, and dogs then suffer as a result of overcrowding and competition for the little food there is, as well as lack of veterinary care. The local councils had taken to using strychnine in an attempt to control dog numbers, but this is an outdated, cruel and completely ineffective method of stray population control. After a round of poisoning, dog numbers simply increase back to their steady state as remaining dogs rebreed.

I learnt so much about charity work and running an 'Animal Birth Control' or ABC centre, as well as seeing first hand the degree of poverty which exists in many third world countries (Nepal is the second poorest country in the world according to recent statistics). One of the main problems associated with such a large stray dog population is the transmission of rabies to both dogs and humans (most commonly children). In areas where successful ABC programmes are running, the rabies infection rate in the local population has decreased from a significant level to virtually zero, so there is a direct benefit for the local people too.

I could write a hundred stories on my time in this charming small country, but I wanted to share the tale of one special little puppy with you, my Momo.

Kathmandu Animal Treatment Centre (KAT centre) neuters around 10,000 animals each year, employing eight full-time staff who work incredibly long hours. And yet they are only able to deal with a small fraction of the city's stray dog problem.

KAT centre's operating facilities are geared toward neutering and minor surgeries. The centre policy is that we had to put to sleep any animals suffering from very serious ailments which required more intensive care than KAT could provide. It might sound like a harsh policy, but the scale of the street dog problem in Kathmandu is so great that they had to 'be cruel to be kind'. Or to phrase it differently, the needs of the many are greater than the needs of the few, and as with all charities, they are working with limited funding.

When Momo (I named her after a type of dumpling eaten by locals), came into KAT centre with a broken leg, we all knew that we should really let her go there and then. But myself, and my colleagues at KAT centre, are only human, and every now and then, you meet an animal that seems so special that you feel you must try for them. As vets, we have to be wary of allowing sentimentality to cloud our professional judgement. If you love animals, then in my experience, the process of decision-making does not in fact always get easier over the years. Experience helps us so much, but personally, I never wish to lose my compassion and consideration for the individual whilst doing what's best for the greater good. It's a hard, nigh on impossible, balance to strike. I know how to switch off my emotions and compassion – I had to do this for four years in farm animal practice, where money takes on equal importance to animal welfare. But it is not how I wish to live my professional life.

Momo was the loveliest black and white collie cross pup. She was about four months old when she was brought in. She was quite thin, because she couldn't compete for food with the other dogs due to her broken leg, but her coat shone and she still smelt of 'clean puppy' (dog owners amongst you will understand what I mean by this!). Her tail was set to 'hyperwag' permanently, which was quite unbalancing for her as she hobbled on three legs! She was obviously very used to interacting with humans. In Nepal, having a pet is the reserve of the rich. But local families will often consider the street dogs of their area as part of their community and look after them by way of throwing them scraps and allowing them to sleep in outbuildings. Very often, the children in particular will form close bonds with the street dogs – children and dogs seem to have an affinity with one another the world over!

The dog handling staff at KAT told me that, in order for the children (who had been caring for her since she broke her leg two days previously) to hand Momo over to KAT centre staff, they had had to promise to return her safely. Poor Momo was in quite a bad way by then, her leg was hanging limp and every time it moved, it was clearly very painful for her. It was obvious that this type of fracture would not heal without surgical intervention.

Sanne – a dutch vet student also volunteering at KAT – took Momo to the prep room so we could examine her further. Sanne and I discussed euthanasia, during a careful discussion on Momo's options. We both agreed to take the next step and X-ray Momo's broken leg to ascertain how bad the damage was. Certain types of fracture were repairable with simple equipment and others were not. Neither of us wanted to put this lovely pup to sleep, even though, every week, we had to euthanase several animals for similar reasons.

The only X-ray machine we had access to was far across the city. Sanne had accompanied animals there previously. There was always a long wait and the X-rays were not of prime quality, but we needed an X-ray before we could decide whether we were able to operate on Momo or not. So we bandaged the fractured leg with a splint and set off across the city in the KAT van, with Momo carefully balanced on our knees to help support her over the bumpy roads.

The X-ray 'parlour', as I would call it, comprised a tiny corridor that led straight in from the hectic street. The space was made even smaller by a reception desk and six waiting-room chairs, positioned halfway down. A door opened to an even smaller room that only just seemed big enough to house the giant, ancient, cumbersome X-ray machine.

We carried Momo up to the reception desk. This was a walk in clinic, which means people can just turn up to be X-rayed and we had to wait two and a half hours before they were ready for Momo. I wasn't too worried about the wait because I had given Momo some long lasting and strong pain relief that morning, and she was quite comfortable. The other patients looked on bemused as we sat in the queue, and they smiled shyly as I photographed Momo waiting with them for her turn to be X-rayed.

When we were called in, I carefully got out the anaesthetic injection that I had brought to sedate Momo for the X-ray. I had placed an intravenous catheter in her leg before we left so that I could do this quickly. In the UK, we very seldom X-ray animals without sedation or general anaesthesia unless they are very placid or unwell, and so will lie still without being held by someone. Momo was not this type of patient! Britain has strict radiation safety laws in place to protect our staff from the serious effects of overexposure to X-ray radiation. So I was horrified when the radiographer asked his assistant to pin Momo down so that he could take the X-ray!

"No, no," I cried and rushed forward with the sedative, gesticulating towards the catheter in Momo's leg. They looked at me with a bemused smile on their lips. So I gave Momo the sedative and she relaxed beautifully, lying in a perfect position for the X-ray without anyone having to stand by the X-ray beam to hold her. The assistant didn't even have gloves or a protective apron, he was prepared to stand holding her with his bare hands – it was unbelievable to me! Next, I had to struggle to get everyone out of the room as the X-ray was taken – they obviously weren't used to this either! At least, I was able to establish a protocol for the KAT staff if they had to take another animal for X-rays, although I hate to think about the poor radiographer's assistant and how much exposure he must suffer on a regular basis.

The X-ray came out well – after another hour's wait, of course! It showed Momo had a simple fracture of the mid shaft of her humerus. The word 'simple' here does not mean it would be easy to repair, it simply means that there were no extra fragments or complications. But it did mean that it was actually repairable, with some basic equipment.

We visited a local vet who we discovered had a small collection of bone plates. The vet had to go up to his loft to find the plate! Orthapaedic instruments, it seems, are like gold dust in Nepal. Dr Thapa proudly showed us his small collection of instruments, and I got the distinct impression he hadn't actually been able to use them very often. But we were incredibly grateful that he lent us a drill and some instruments as well as selling us the bone plate (though he did request the plate back after it had been removed once the bone had healed!).

I made a phone call to a veterinary orthopaedic specialist I knew back home to ask for some advice. I described the fracture in detail to him and we discussed repair options. Fortunately, Sanne had brought with her a very good orthopaedic text to study for her exams. It told me quite clearly that repairs of the humerus were difficult and had a high risk of nerve damage (if the nerve had not already been damaged by the fracture itself). But the orthopaedic surgeon reassured me by pointing out that the surgery was really Momo's only chance of survival as this type of fracture would not heal without intervention, and amputation of a street dog's leg was not a viable option.

On the morning of the surgery, I felt very nervous. Whenever I operate, I feel that each little life is so precious and sacred that I am afraid of doing harm. I would never have admitted this fear to anyone as a new graduate in case people thought I was not suitable for the job – that I wasn't 'tough' enough. For routine, straightforward procedures, this just manifests for me as extreme care and respect for the animal – I try and treat each pet I operate on as I would if it were my own or even myself! But for more complicated procedures, especially if I have not performed them before, I can often feel quite afraid. The trick is not to let this affect my surgery skills and I have learnt to do this over time.

We sweated for a long time over Momo's leg in the hot, humid theatre, which seemed to catch all of the day's sun like a greenhouse. I carefully followed the instructions in the book and my own notes I had made whilst talking to the specialist. But the fractured bone ends were very difficult to reposition correctly. The muscles around most broken bones contract and it can be very difficult to 'reduce' (i.e. reset) a fracture accurately. My arms were aching and I wondered if I would have to abandon my efforts and put Momo to sleep after all. We had all wanted to help Momo so much, but that isn't always enough when dealing with nature. I was literally at the point of my last attempt to reduce the fracture, when the bones clunked beautifully into place, allowing me to tighten the screws on the bone plate to stabilise it.

We all let out a huge sigh of relief before I sutured Momo's muscle layers and skin as quickly as possible. She had been under anaesthetic for some time now and we wanted to get her woken up quickly.

Despite the lengthy procedure, Momo recovered well from the anaesthetic and her little tail was soon wagging again. We took her up to the X-ray parlour again the next day and the 'post op' X-rays showed a successful fracture repair.

Over the next few days, Momo started using the leg more and more and we were very pleased with her progress. I had to return home about one week after the surgery and I was heartbroken to leave Momo behind, but the staff at KAT promised to keep me up to date with her progress, and I felt very happy to think that she would return to her home with the children who loved her so much. The plan was for the new KAT centre surgeon to remove the plate after one month and then Momo would be free to return to her 'community'. I received regular reports of her antics, running round at the centre and terrorising all the other patients!

I would love to finish the story there, as Momo was doing so well after the op and was so happy. But sometimes life has some very sad twists and this is as much a part of our job as are the happier tales. Poor Momo got poorly about one month after the operation. She had a raging temperature and she developed signs of brain disease. She was diagnosed with Canine Distemper Virus, even though we had vaccinated her, as was Centre policy, on admission to KAT. This can happen, although it is very rare. Her condition worsened quickly and staff at the KAT centre decided that euthanasia was necessary on welfare grounds and also to prevent disease from spreading to other animals. It was a devastating blow to all of us – for Momo to have come through so much and then to succumb to Distemper virus. It seemed so very unfair.

We are left with such little comfort after cases like this. They happen in general practice too – when unbelievable bad luck intervenes and causes great difficulty and loss.

My acceptance of these situations lies in knowing that we did our best and treated the animal with compassion; and also, in promising myself not to give up or become cynical or negative because something like this has happened. Otherwise, I might miss a chance at helping an animal, or a person in need through focusing on my own pain and disappointment. Good things happen – amazing, excellent things that inspire and encourage us. And bad things happen – terrible, unlucky, sad things that disappoint and frighten us. But we can never predict fully how anything might turn out – just as in life – and we have to keep trying and remember how precious the simple things are.

It might sound sentimental, but I think of Momo often – of her innocent doggy joy in simply being alive, her perpetually wagging tail, and her little wet nose that always smudged my glasses. She brought a lot of joy into many peoples' lives in her short life. Through the experience of performing a new surgery on her when I was so afraid of getting it wrong, she taught me to have more trust in my own abilities. In turn, the lessons I learned from Momo's surgery – the experience and confidence it gave me – have benefited all of the other animals that I treat. Rightly or wrongly, I believe that every little thing that happens has some purpose, even if we can't see it ourselves, and this helps me to get on with my job and help as many people and animals as I can.

Mhairi Cameron

African Days – The Cowardly Hippo

The two years I spent in practice in Kenya were amongst my most interesting. They started with a bang: on my first day I was bitten by a dog suspected of being rabid.

Vaccination soon after exposure prevents the development of the dreaded symptoms so I lost no time in organising my inoculations.

At that time the vaccinations were comprised of fourteen injections, given one a day into the abdominal fat. Each was horribly painful and elicited a reaction the size of a hen's egg. Of course I had less abdominal fat in those days than I have now, so by the end of the course there were three or four layers of reactions superimposed on one another and I staggered about my duties agonised, hunched up like Quasimodo.

I lived on a farm close to Lake Nakuru, home to a million pink flamingos, often depicted in the Kenya travel brochures. Water from the lake flowed to a dam on our farm and at night hippo wandered up this waterway to graze on the young "mealie" sprouts, causing colossal damage to the crops and fences. The farm owner, a wonderfully colourful character, was driven to the end of her tether and was forever threatening to have the hippos shot.

However when it came to the push she always contrived to relent and I almost had cause to regret this, as I will now relate.

That year a combined Cape Universities rugby team came on tour. Modesty prevents me from saying that our local team was one of the best in Kenya, but I can say that we gave them a close run. The excellent game was followed by the usual party and towards the early hours of the morning I offered to conduct our guests to the lake and show them the flamingos by moonlight.

We parked our cars as close as possible and blundered down to the water's edge. I carried a hockey stick by way of support and after our night of unbridled revelry you might say it provided a welcome element of stability.

Suddenly, no more than five metres ahead of us, a colossal, tank-like animal reared up out of the undergrowth. In an instant I was as sober as a judge and in another I took off like the proverbial bat out of hell.

It is amazing what suitable incentives will do for athleticism and I am convinced that over a hundred metres I would have beaten Linford Christie decisively, even giving him a few metres start out of the blocks.

I remember clutching my hockey stick tightly as I ran, determined to lash out at the animal if it caught up and to sell my life dearly.

Luckily this cowardly beast was as afraid of us as we were of him and he fled almost as quickly in the opposite direction!

Leonard Black

The Last Straw – An Incident I'd Rather Forget

Perhaps the funniest incident of my career happened in the serious context of an international scientific conference.

Research work is not the dramatic occupation that many people imagine it to be, and the brilliant scientist who suddenly thinks up cures for cancer and CJD dwell only in the imagination of the "Eureka, I have it" school of Hollywood script writers.

In reality it is a slow, repetitive occupation where the main requirement is stubborn determination to pursue an investigation to it's bitter end, and the usual outcome is the addition of a tiny drop of information to the vast ocean of previous knowledge. From one day to the next it is the most frustrating work imaginable. However, its very frustrations are what make the job fascinating and there is nothing quite so exciting as seeing a tableau unfold before you, bit by bit, with exquisite slowness. If you manage to achieve what you set out to do the most wonderful feeling of euphoria follows and you float on a cloud whenever you think about the scrap of information that you yourself contributed to the scientific world.

But the laboratory results are only half the battle for you have yet to publicise your findings. This can be done by sending a report about your work to one of the scientific journals or by giving a talk at an international conference attended by those interested in your topic. This brings me to the subject of my story.

I was giving a talk on the vaccination of cattle against foot and mouth disease at a conference in Tel Aviv. It was a humid, Mediterranean day and it was my misfortune to be speaking in the middle of the afternoon, by which time the audience was flagging from the information-packed talks that had preceded my own at ten-minute intervals since early morning.

My turn was to follow the tea break and I had the bright idea of illustrating the talk with both transparency slides and overhead projections so that I could show different aspects of the topic simultaneously on two adjacent screens. This is not a usual procedure. In theory it was a nice concept but in practice it turned out an unmitigated disaster.

In the first place the projectionist was about five minutes late returning from tea. 'Five minutes' does not sound long but with everyone hot and impatient it seemed like an eternity. Next, when both the projectors were switched on we found that the shadow of the one impinged on the projection thrown by the other, so everything had to be moved and focused again.

At long last I was rigged up with a microphone clipped to my shirt, the lights were dimmed and we were ready to start. But even then the tale of woe went on. At that stage my pack of carefully arranged acetate projection sheets spilled to the ground and transparent as they were, it was almost impossible to see them on the dark carpet in the muted light.

So there I was, hot and bothered myself, on hands and knees in the semi darkness, trying to feel about the floor for the almost invisible bits of plastic in front of a crowd of impatient, tired people.

Quite forgetting the microphone that hovered a few inches below my chin and speaking under my breath, I gave vent to all my pent up exasperation. Or rather, I thought it was under my breath. Instead the microphones blared out my words to the furthest corners of the auditorium and I heard myself telling the august assembly of learned scientists, "Good God, this is a prize fuck-up."

For a moment I stood aghast in the quietness that ensued and then the whole place exploded into a most tumultuous roar of laughter. They laughed … they laughed … they were falling about in their seats laughing while I could only wait, grinning sheepishly, for it all to subside. At last, after what seemed an eternity, it did so and the best round of applause I have ever received followed my talk. I would like to think that this was in appreciation of my brilliant scientific findings but somehow I doubt it.

Leonard Black

Chapter 6 – More Vets' Funny Stories

The Lost Bat

A client came into the consult room carrying a small cardboard box. I hated to see cardboard boxes, especially small ones, as it usually meant that there was a small creature in it, either a hamster or a guinea pig or even a pet rat. I preferred to see dogs and cats rather than small furries or exotics. Thankfully I have not yet had to see a pet spider or a snake and I hope I never have to! In my opinion these are best off seen by an exotics specialist.

In this case it turned out to my surprise to be a small bat. Being a rural practice there are occasions when the public bring in sick or injured wildlife, most of which we end up euthanasing for welfare reasons. The client carefully picked up the bat with his bare hands and placed it on the consult room table. Having graduated from Edinburgh University I remembered there was some press about a man contracting rabies from a group of wild bats in Scotland somewhere. Unfortunately I never forgot this snippet of press and in my memory I see a bat as a possible rabies risk! Having never handled a bat before I did not feel that the thin latex gloves I had available were thick enough should it bite, so I picked up the thick anti-cat-bite 'gauntlets' that we had for vicious and evil cats. In hindsight this was a little extreme on my part but one can never be too careful – we come into contact with all sorts of species' bugs on a regular basis. The saying is that vets must be immune to everything going otherwise we'd be ill all the time. The bat was no bigger than the length of my thumb so it did look a little ridiculous on my gauntlets! I wasn't expecting it to be so small. After holding it for a few minutes hoping it wouldn't jump off (I couldn't hold on to it any tighter for fear of squashing it with my clumsy gloves) I replaced it back in the box. The bat looked fairly lifeless, remaining still the whole time.

The client laughed at me fumbling around with my gloves, so I explained that bats could carry rabies. He looked a little surprised and I think he realised then that he should have been a little more careful when handling wildlife. Many of the public when picking up sick wildlife never think of the potential consequences of being bitten or scratched and contracting a bug of some sorts and they never think to wear gloves. For example hedgehogs can carry a lot of ringworm, which can readily pass to humans and other species. Well OK I'll use that as my defence for my excessive gloves, which my colleague also found very amusing. "You won't get rabies" she retorted. But I'd rather be safe than sorry.

The bat had been found soaking wet near a pond and was thought to have crash landed, half drowning itself and the client agreed to leaving the bat with us for nursing care but said he would like to take it home to release where he found it.

My task of the morning was to find out more about bats. Having phoned around a couple of practices I found a nurse in another practice who regularly cared for injured bats. I took her advice and nursed the bat giving it a soft paste type of dog food – normally used for recovering dogs – that is kind to the guts. I cut the bottom off a plastic cup from our 'water at work' container, placed some food in the bottom and now with my latex gloves on I held it up to the bat's face – the food was nearly as big as the bat! The bat ate and I was fascinated to see its tiny mouth opening against the massive disc of food. I thought to myself, "You're frightened of that!" No wonder I got laughed at earlier.

I left the bat for a few more hours in its cardboard box in a dog cage. When I returned to check on it again, to my surprise the bat had much improved and this time when I carefully lifted the lid of the box it flew straight at me. I fell backwards – it was so fast moving. I flapped my arms around like an idiot trying to get the bat out of my face. Finally I caught sight of its rapid, jerky movements just to catch a glimpse of the bat leaving through the back door for its return to the wild! I ran to the back door, which was open, as the boss just happened to be sorting his car out. I looked around, trying to see it, but bats move so quickly it was nowhere to be seen.

I had just lost a bat – what was I going to say to the client who had wanted to take it home for his young daughter to release? I put off for another couple of hours, managing to keep myself busy doing paperwork in the office.

"Have you rung the client about the bat yet?"

"No I haven't," I replied, "I haven't worked out what to say yet."

"Just tell him you lost it."

I plucked up the courage to ring the client and explained what had happened, finishing with "in fact it got so much better that it flew at me and as a result got past me and out of the door." To my relief the client burst out laughing and wanted more details. So I explained how it had got better throughout the day and how it must just have been hypothermic, it had eaten food and how it had flown in my face.

Anonymous

Hope

It was the kind of call that every on-call vet dreads. After a long Saturday stitching up cut pads, tending to fly-struck rabbits and endlessly cleaning up after a vomiting in-patient, all I wanted to do was get home and have a bite to eat.

Inevitably, just as I was locking up, my mobile phone went off again. Hope, a nine-month-old Golden Retriever, was poorly. She had been sick on and off for 24 hours but could no longer keep water down and was very out of sorts.

Her owner was clearly concerned and in the circumstances I felt I had no option but to at least examine her. She arrived at the surgery looking very forlorn, and a brief examination revealed all the signs of an animal starting to go into shock. Moreover when I felt her tummy, there was a large painful lump right in the middle of her abdomen. I realised with a sinking feeling that this was not something which would right itself with a few pills.

I admitted Hope for intravenous fluid therapy and further investigation. She seemed a little brighter on her drip but X-rays failed to reveal anything more than the aforementioned lump in her tummy. I was left with no choice but to perform an exploratory laparotomy operation. As I explored the depths of her abdominal cavity, the problem soon became apparent – a length of her small intestine was bruised, angry and distended with a firm obstruction. Carefully I opened the offending stretch of bowel to expose a dark green fabric structure. As I gently teased it through the incision, it gradually unfurled, revealing itself to be the most enormous pair of Y-fronts I have ever seen! The owner was a young lady who lived alone who claimed never to have seen the pants, or to know anyone who might wear them. Their origin remains a mystery to this day, but I am pleased to report that Hope made a full and rapid recovery and has never since been known to eat underwear.

Anonymous

Squiggles

Squiggles, was a three-month-old kitten who paid the price for youthful exuberance and extreme nosiness. From the moment his new owners took him home, he had apparently been fond of sticking his nose into places it didn't belong.

We received a telephone call from his distressed owners one morning after they had found him with his head stuck through a hole in one end of a low bench seat.

They had initially requested a home visit, but were unwilling to pay the increased fee that such a visit would incur, so instead chose to saw off the end support of the bench and bring it to the surgery with the kitten in situ!!

Squiggles seemed quite unperturbed by the whole affair, standing quietly on the examination table with his neck supported by his somewhat unorthodox collar. Despite his calmness, it was deemed too dangerous to try and saw the wood off from directly round his neck, so with a generous helping of lubricant gel we set about trying to get him back out the way he came.

After much huffing and puffing on my part, and some protestations from Squiggles about his now somewhat soggy fur, we eventually freed him – he popped back through the hole apparently none the worse for wear, albeit rather bedraggled.

This would have been the happy end to the story, but for the fact that his owners had neglected to remove the remainder of the bench and its associated support from the garden and so Squiggles returned back to the surgery later the same day, wearing another wooden collar, and still unfazed by his predicament. Fortunately the lubricant worked again and this time his owners were careful to remove any such temptations from his environment!

Anonymous

An Embarrassing Consult

"What can I do for you Reverend?"

"Well I noticed the other day that he had a lump between, well, hmm, his bits," said Reverend Matthews.

I examined the dog but could not find a lump anywhere, "Where exactly is the lump?"

"Right between his balls and his 'widgie'," he replied. (Why is it that members of the public always refer to such things in this way, I mean what's wrong with the technical terms of penis and testicles?!)

"Well, there's nothing there now."

"Well it's not there all the time, I only noticed it when I was towel drying Ben after he'd been swimming," replied the Reverend.

I suddenly understood what he was referring to and wondered how I could word this in a professional manner without blushing.

"It's okay, that's quite normal," I said patiently, "It sounds as though he's just getting a bit excited when he's being towel dried, and well, hmm, he's a male dog... you see?"

I think the Reverend got the message as he started to look a little flustered. He quickly thanked me for looking at his dog and turned to go out the door. I followed him back to reception, as he was the only client in.

"How much do I owe you?" said the Reverend.

I looked at Ruth, the receptionist, "No charge for that," I said, "the dog just gets a bit excited."

Ruth, who knew the dog had come in to have his 'lumps' examined, quickly got what I meant and smiled kindly to the Reverend, "It's okay, I think you've paid with embarrassment!"

Anonymous

Doh!!!

I recently had a consult with Mrs Rose and her very sweet looking Bearded Collie cross called Jack. Mrs Rose looked very proud of Jack as I called them into the consult room, and commented on what a lovely boy he was. He was so cute it looked like butter wouldn't melt in his mouth.

As I examined Jack for his annual vaccinations, however, he started to grumble and growl at me. As it was my standard procedure for this situation, I politely asked the owner if she would mind me muzzling Jack to err on the side of caution. I always ask an owner first, before muzzling an animal, as some owners can have a peculiar aversion to this and can be quite offended if I muzzle their animal without checking it out with them first.

It was a good job I asked, because Mrs Rose looked upset and immediately stated in no uncertain terms that a muzzle was not necessary for her Jack. He wouldn't ever snap or bite, and she was perfectly capable of holding him for me.

Well, that was me told, I thought, and decided that discretion was going to be the better part of valour in this case. So I carefully continued examining Jack. Unfortunately, Jack's naughtiness escalated and he did indeed start turning his head to try and nip me. Obviously, in such situations, I do not wish to be bitten myself, but I feel an even greater concern for the health and safety of my clients (I am less likely to sue myself for loss of digits than they are, amongst other reasons).

Generally, my stock phrase in such cases would be, "Oh, I am really sorry but I think we are going to have to pop a muzzle on Jack as I don't want him to give you a nip by mistake whilst he's aiming at me." For some unknown reason, however, on this occasion, I used a phrase I have never used before,

"Oh, I am really sorry but we ought to pop a muzzle on Jack now. I don't want him to bite off all your fingers!" As I said this, I noted what a peculiar phrase this was for me to use and felt slightly sheepish for having said it (not half as sheepish as I was about to feel however).

The lady stiffened perceptibly and I thought I must have offended her by suggesting that 'her Jack' might do such a thing. Jack seemed quite offended too and he tried to launch himself off the table several times. As I went to help the owner to hold him still, she altered her grip, and her right hand, which had previously been hidden by Jack's fur, came into full view. I couldn't believe it because I saw that her right hand was completely 'finger and thumb-less'. No more than half an inch of finger or thumb protruded from each knuckle. To make matters worse, I was so stunned by the retrospective inappropriateness of my previous comment that my eyes were fixed to her deformed hand like glue. I was speechless for a moment and blushed scarlet before I opened my mouth to apologise. But after standing with my mouth gaping for a few moments, I decided that perhaps bringing the subject up might offend Mrs Rose even further.

So I hastily gave Jack his booster injection and turned back to my computer to write up my notes, or rather, to hide my still scarlet face. Poor Mrs Rose, I thought over and over again. How could I be so insensitive?

As I turned back round to Mrs Rose to complete the consult in my usual manner, by opening the door and saying something to round things off, Mrs Rose had a beaming smile on her face.

"Thank you for being so kind to Jack," she said, still grinning, and then, tapping my arm with her fingerless hand, she chuckled. "Don't worry! You are absolutely right – I don't want to lose any more fingers!" And we both laughed. I wondered afterwards if my subconscious had subliminally noticed Mrs Rose's lack of fingers, hence why I had used such an uncharacteristic phrase, or if it was just an unlucky coincidence. Either way, I was very relieved that I hadn't upset poor Mrs Rose.

Mhairi Cameron

The Donkey

When working Saturday mornings at our practice there was only one vet and the receptionist/nurse on duty so rather than booking in consultations and visits everyone was told to ring before coming in just in case the vet had gone out elsewhere. It was my turn on the rota to do this particular Saturday. To start with a few people rang up to ask if they could bring their pets in. I noticed however that after my first consult, the receptionist had booked in a visit for me to see a donkey. This would not be my favourite of visits as I'd had some bad experiences with equine (horse) clients in the past so I asked if there were any further details given on the phone. Paul, the receptionist wasn't really sure what it was about, all he had been told was that the donkey was not well, and the owners weren't sure if it was in foal or not and what if the donkey didn't have enough milk like their last one. I replied to Paul, that I would ring them before I left, as I didn't have a clue what I needed in my car from the confusing and mismatching information available. I had to wait until I had finished seeing a few more clients who were already on their way down to the surgery before I could set off for the donkey.

I worried about it all morning, especially when I realised that the owner had another donkey, which an ex-partner had been out to see, which he had sent on to a referral centre for a possible Caesarean as he couldn't get the foal out. The owner was not happy about the situation although I didn't know the specifics of why, just bits of gossip I had picked up from ear wagging a conversation a few days ago. When I'd finished the consults, I looked at the book again and no the visit hadn't been cancelled and there was no one else in to go and do it. I couldn't put off any longer. I phoned the owner for more information but despite my best efforts I couldn't untangle the history of what was wrong either so I had to depart knowing only that the donkey was "just not right".

I found the place without difficulty and the owners – husband and wife – met me at the car. It was a hot day so I didn't put my waterproofs on, just wellies. I examined the donkey, starting as usual with its head. The wife continued to talk and asked me if the donkey was going to foal. However when I asked her when it was due she replied that she didn't know. The husband remained silent. He just stood there listening intently, letting his wife do all the talking. I had a feel of the donkey's abdomen and sure enough I could feel the solid lump of a foal through her sides. To my surprise the owner then said, "You'd better put your hand in, see if there's anything there." She also started to explain about how the other pet donkey had foaled two weeks ago and had not shown any signs of foaling, and how my colleague had been out to see her. So I carefully placed my lubricated hand into the vagina of the donkey and to my surprise her cervix was fully open. It was strange, as the donkey had made no attempts to strain or push at all. I could feel the foal on the other side of a thickened membrane. I reported my findings to the owner, who kept talking the whole time whilst her husband still stood motionless. My mind turned over and over again. It felt like I was feeling the foal through the uterus wall and if I tried to pull it, the wall seemed to come with it. It felt very strange indeed. I couldn't seem to manage to feel the foal without feeling the wall too. Her cervix was definitely open so I couldn't understand it. I thought harder and finally came to realise that it was just the placenta but a lot thicker than I was used to feeling in other animals.

I had only calved cows and lambed sheep before and their placentae were different to that of an equine and are much thinner. I remember now studying the placentae in vet school anatomy lessons. In principle foaling a donkey is the same as calving a cow. However horses and donkeys usually foal unassisted and quickly (within 20 minutes) so it is not very often a vet gets the opportunity to foal one. I boldly put my fingers through the thick membrane and broke it. I could now feel the foal properly, 'phew', and began to put ropes on its legs to help pull it out. However the head went back when I pulled and it was obvious that I needed a head snare on (a piece of rope round the back of the head to keep the head pulled in line with the legs). This was easier said than done. To place the head snare I had to put the rope over its head and behind its ears. But this was a donkey and not a calf; its ears were very long and laid back against its neck. However after a struggle, reaching and pulling forwards a mile of donkey ear, I finally managed to get the snare in place.

"Quick," shouted the owner to her friend who had just pulled up in her car, "the foal is nearly out!" With a pull the foal came out followed by all the fluids, soaking me. How I wished I'd worn my waterproofs! The placenta followed (thankfully as it can cause serious complications if it is retained for too long) and I looked at it now actually seeing and remembering the differences in types of placenta.

The foal coughed and spluttered, shaking its head with its ears flapping and splashing us in foetal fluids, as if I wasn't already wet enough. The owner and friend were delighted with the foal and stood watching, commenting on how cute it was. The donkey licked the foal's fur as the long-legged lanky creature struggled on to its knees. I was happy to see the mother taking a good interest in her newborn foal, which was eager to get to its feet. Feeling relieved that the foaling was over, I collected my equipment and washed my ropes before leaving the field.

As we walked across the courtyard to the house to wash my hands before leaving we discussed the milk for the foal. The owners were concerned, as the previous donkey had also foaled in a similar way (not showing any signs of foaling, also having no milk) and her foal had died. I agreed that they should supplement this foal with milk substitute. It was the husband's turn to speak this time.

"Oh, have you got a tit on you?!" he said without thinking. I laughed to myself – typical bloke.

"No, sorry, you'll have to collect a dummy teat to feed the foal with from the surgery later," I replied. He went red as he realised what he had just said, and his wife just laughed.

I left the place with a great feeling – I had just successfully foaled a donkey for the first and probably last time and I felt privileged to have done so. I was very satisfied that I had done a good job for the client and I hope the client appreciated my achievement. In the end it turned out to be a challenging but very satisfying visit.

Helen Woodvine

Chapter 7 – Vets' Fears

Smith Hilltop

The phone rang, jolting me awake from a light sleep in my warm cosy bed (one never sleeps as well when on call). The sound of my mobile belted out, increasing in volume with each ring. I shot up, fumbling around on the floor, trying to find my phone before it rang off. My heart rate rocketed, partly from waking up so quickly, and partly from the shock of hearing the on-call mobile tune that I now dread so much.

"Hello?" I said, trying to hide my sleepy voice.

"Hello Jane. It's been a quiet night so far hasn't it?" It was Mary looking after the phones that night. As usual, she started off with pleasantries, trying to allow me time to come round and realise what was going on. She was experienced at manning the phones and having to wake vets up from their sleep.

"I have a call for you."

Yes, get on with it, just tell me! I thought, rather grumpily. As a recent graduate, I hung off her every word waiting to see what the call was. It could be a calving, a sick dog, a maggoty rabbit, a horse with colic – anything!

"Smith, Hilltop has got two difficult lambings for you."

Mary had arranged for me to meet them at the surgery. I looked at my watch – it was 11.30pm. I must have been asleep for less than half an hour.

A sheep, I thought. *That's not too bad, I can cope with a lambing*. I had enjoyed my lambing experience at vet school and felt happy to do a sheep Caesarean if required. I had done the first couple of the season last week already, plus several the previous season.

I quickly got dressed, and rushed to the toilet, as I didn't know when I would next get a chance to go! It was a cold night, drizzling with rain, but I lived close to the surgery so it didn't take long to get there. My partner – John, came with me for moral support.

We arrived at the surgery before the farmer so I checked his file on the computer. He had been to the vet's for quite a few lambings already this year, and in the past for a lot of calvings. I noted that he had been to our other branch surgery recently with three sheep Caesareans in one day! I thought that was a lot. As vets, we recommend that farmers don't breed an animal in such a way that it can't give birth naturally.

I heard a voice outside, "Hello?" I called out as I walked briskly to the back door.

"Hello." I said again. "Two lambings? Would you like to get them both out for me?" I recognised at this point that I had seen these farmers before; they were two brothers who always seemed to be arguing about something! A strange pair, by all accounts, as I had heard the office staff talking about them. They were well known in the neighbouring town for other reasons. Apparently all the local bridges had their names spray-painted on them with reference to an affair of some sort (it's a small world here). However I had not had direct dealings with them before, so I tried not to feel too apprehensive despite their somewhat jaded reputation.

"Just one at a time, my dear. I think they will both need a 'Caesar'," replied the taller brother with the long chin.

"Oh?" I said, "I see you had three 'Caesars' in one day last week?"

It was at this point that the events that night started to turn and the taller brother responded by gruffly mumbling "I see you've done your homework."

I had thought it unusual to have so many Caesarean sections in one day, and in my ignorance, it had fascinated me enough to comment on it out of interest. But he seemed less impressed.

The other brother had lifted the first ewe onto the table in the lambing room. Freezing cold, I put some lubricant onto my hand in order to feel inside the ewe's womb to see what the problem was.

Her cervix was fully dilated and the lamb was presented normally. However, her pelvis was very small and the lamb was very large. Whilst I was carefully examining around the lamb, to decide if a Caesarean section was indeed necessary, the ewe 'pushed' and a sudden spurt of blood ran past my hand and onto the floor. The blood did not continue.

"What's that?" shouted the shorter brother with dark hair.

"I don't know where it's from yet," I replied honestly. It was not possible that I had caused any internal damage because I had not tried to pull the lamb with any ropes or tension. I didn't know where the blood was from and my mind raced, trying to work it out. It seemed strange, but I couldn't feel any tear in the uterus or ruptured vessels. I quickly confirmed the two brothers' suspicions that the ewe needed a Caesarean, because the lamb was large, her pelvis was small and she was, after all, a 'Beltex' (a breed notorious for being unable to pass a lamb).

My partner clipped the sheep for me as I quickly prepared the equipment and scrubbed my hands clean.

"Aren't you going to sedate her?"

"No," I replied. "It would be better if you could just sit with her quietly, she won't feel anything as I've given her a local anaesthetic block and she'll be better able to let the lambs suckle straight afterwards and less likely to lie on them."

"But they sedate them at the other branch!"

I didn't know that the vets in the other branch gave sedation for sheep Caesareans, but on previous discussion with my boss I knew that he preferred not to. So I held my ground and said, "She'll be okay if you sit on the table next to her and hold on to her head so she can't get up." I had already tied the ewe's back legs to the table as was standard practice, so she would be unable to kick me or make an exit anyway.

I carefully started to cut through the skin on the ewe's flank.

"You'll have to make your hole a little bigger than that my dear!" One of the brothers sneered.

I was too busy concentrating on what I was doing to take any notice of him, but my partner stood there prickling with anger. He had already taken a disliking to the inappropriate comments made by the taller brother.

I quickly found the uterus – the lamb was in the horn furthest away from me, which made the Caesarean a lot more technically difficult. Still, the brothers took it in turns to make unrelentless snide comments the whole way through the operation, which was already extremely difficult and stressful (I now know that this was the most difficult Caesar I had ever done).

I struggled to get any part of the lamb to the surface.

"Why can't you find it?"

"It's awkward because it's on the other side." I wished they would give me some time to work. Eventually, I was able to get the lamb up and cut into the uterus to pull the first leg out.

"Why are you pulling the front leg and not the back leg? It was coming forwards!"

"Well, because it's all I can get hold of and it happens to be a front leg! It doesn't matter which way it comes out, it just happens to be lying that way," I responded, trying to be as patient as possible.

Finally, I got the lamb out, but it was stillborn.

"Why is it dead?"

"All I can think of is that spurt of blood earlier was somehow the navel cord rupturing and the lamb must have died there and then," I replied honestly. This was the only explanation I could think of.

Silence.

The shorter brother turned away from us, leaning against the wall with his head in his arm, as if he could not cope with the fact that the lamb was dead. The other lamb came out without a problem and was alive.

John held the uterus together for me, which, to my horror, was shrinking so fast back into the ewe that I started to panic. I had to stitch rapidly, though this became increasingly more difficult as the ewe's uterus contracted. The brothers' presence was making me increasingly nervous and uncomfortable. I stabbed my finger several times with the needle, drawing blood, and the thread seemed to keep on tangling. Still their unpleasant comments kept coming, chipping away at me with every criticism imaginable. How I wished it was over and that they would just keep quiet. My hands started to shake uncontrollably – the only time this has ever happened to me through nerves and stress. Beads of sweat ran down my face. I was embarrassed that they could see how much they were getting to me, and I could see the cruel satisfaction they took in watching me. John watched on, wishing that he could do more to help.

Finally it was done. An hour and a half had passed and I was tired and stressed, I really couldn't face another sheep Caesar. My mind ran away, wondering if Peter the boss could come and help.

"Right we'll get the other one out now," they said, not allowing me a moment's reprise.

Begrudgingly I examined the next ewe, also a Beltex. To my disgust it was exactly the same, another big lamb presented normally and the ewe fully dilated. Again it was to be a Caesar.

"So are you going to sedate this one now then?" One of the brothers sniped.

That was it – I couldn't go on.

"I'm not prepared to do another one for you like this, I'll go and phone Peter and he will come and operate for you," I replied and started to walk towards reception for the phone. I could see that the two men were taken aback at this and for the first time there was a pause before anyone spoke.

My partner broke the silence, speaking directly to the two men, "And I'll back her up because I don't like your attitude!" I could tell how upset he was by the tone of his voice.

The frustration of being helpless and watching me shake nervously had eventually got to John and he could not hold back any longer. Whilst I welcomed his support, unfortunately it also provoked the brothers.

The next set of events happened so quickly, I don't even remember exactly what was said but there was a lot of aggressive shouting. The taller brother picked up the ewe and she flew from the table into the trailer without her legs even touching the floor! Had she been a cartoon she would have left her image behind her at the table! Next I saw the smaller brother grab my partner's shirt and push him backwards towards the steel lambing table. John didn't respond and tried to diffuse the situation.

Suddenly I felt very frightened, as I became aware of the tools around us – a scalpel blade, an oxygen bottle in the corner from the day's delivery, which had not been moved and the solid steel table. There was blood and foetal fluids on the floor making it slippery. It was dark outside and no one to hear a shout should it be given. All help seemed so far away. I stepped in between them, putting up my hand to my waist height, "Leave him alone."

The man backed off. "See that dead lamb there? That's worth more to me than …" I don't remember the rest of his sentence. The two brothers hurled abuse at us as they slammed the ramp shut and moved to the vehicle doors to leave. "Look, I'll get Peter to do the surgery." But the brothers ignored me and jumped into their truck. They sped off in a hurry.

I flung my arms around John asking if he was okay. "Ring Peter now," he responded. I acted on his advice and rang Peter straight away. He answered his phone and I explained what had happened, still struggling to hold back the tears and my voice trembling.

"Don't worry, they'll have gone up the road to the other vet's in town. They're not good clients anyway," he said, trying to reassure me.

But he seemed to miss the point a little! The whole experience was extremely frightening and my partner was physically threatened, which had really upset me.

"We'll write them a letter on Monday telling them that if they are going to treat our vets like that then they are not welcome at our practice."

I settled for that and put the phone down. I could not contain my tears any longer as John asked me if I was okay.

I realised that night the importance of safety when we are expected to go and deal with members of the public late at night. We frequently go to a farm or do house visits alone. Most people would never dream of doing such a thing under normal circumstances, indeed it would be considered foolish for any normal young woman to expose herself to such situations. If problems arise, there is no record of where we have attended, other than the phone call and our own notes on the visit (which we make after the visit has taken place). Indeed, if problems arose through the night, no one would be aware of them until the following morning. There is no CCTV at the surgery (just a dummy camera placed as a deterrent to a drunken man who kept fouling in the car park!). That night the dangers were all too real – what if John had fallen? Hit his head on the table behind? What about the scalpel, the oxygen bottle and the other blunt-ended tools?

I felt like I wanted to report the incident to the police, but I did not through fear of the brothers finding out and harassing us further. Next I felt like reporting them to the RSPCA for knowingly breeding animals that cannot give birth without a Caesarean section.

My boss is very laid back and he never did write that letter to the brothers. I was too ashamed to keep reminding him. I didn't want to admit to him just how frightened I had been. In fact, I felt completely unable to discuss it further and ask for more safety measures to be put in place.

When Peter went on a visit to the farm several months later, the two brothers tried to complain about that night. Well informed of the events, my boss told them I didn't do anything wrong – that I did everything exactly as he would have done. With that, Peter told me later, they apologised! However they have never apologised directly to either John or myself. Fortunately, they mainly use the other branch surgery, and I have not had dealings with them since. I would not be happy to see them again either and we have made arrangements for the boss to go should they ring when I am on call. I have also warned my colleagues to be aware of them. It turned out that the brothers had not gone to the practice up the road but had taken the poor ewe straight home and lambed it themselves, killing both the ewe and the lamb in the process.

The events of that night bothered me for some time and I did feel somewhat let down by my boss for not sending that letter. To me it was unacceptable behaviour, which should not be tolerated.

Anonymous

Testing Testing... The Final Straw

I had wanted to be a farm vet ever since I was young. I loved being outside and just about anything to do with farming. Through vet school, I did well in farm animal practical work and I got on well with the farmers. When I started my first job as a mixed but predominantly large animal practitioner, I had worked hard to prove myself amongst the local farmers. After time, however, most of them accepted me and trusted that I could do the job.

Things changed for me when my boss decided to put me through my 'Local Veterinary Inspector' training so I could do my share of the practice's tuberculosis (TB) testing for the (then) 'Ministry of Agriculture, Fisheries and Food'. My colleagues all sympathised with me when I completed the training because, far from giving me new and interesting work to do, as most extra training might, it meant that I would have to spend many full working days on farm, often testing over five hundred cattle per day for exposure to tuberculosis.

In order to perform the test, animals had to be run individually through a crush cage (a large metal crate-like contraption), in order to restrain them, and then we had to clip two areas on their neck with scissors. The skin thickness was carefully measured to a half millimetre with callipers before two injections were given into the skin with an injection gun. The cattle always resented the injections significantly and tended to throw their heads around, making the job difficult and dangerous. There was a high risk of getting an arm caught between the cow and the metal bars of the crush cage.

Testing, as we called it, had to be completed no matter what the weather. Often, we would be outside all day, wet through, freezing cold and always covered in cow muck – a smell you could never get rid of completely! It was a wild affair if young unhandled animals were involved – as the 'heifers and stirks' (young female and male cattle) would be very worked up – panting, sweating, trembling, kicking and trying to jump over barriers which the Health and Safety Executive would have a field day with!

If a farmer was well prepared, with lots of help, then the job could be quite efficient. On less organised farms, the whole affair would be slow and difficult, and you were expected to do a significant amount of manhandling the cattle to keep them moving, as well as conducting the test itself. In a way, this could be good fun, but it was also exhausting when you consider that many of the farmers I had to work with were elderly pensioners (the average age of a farmer in the UK, including school leavers, is fifty nine!). The old saying "there's always one" rings so true when you are trying to get a massive herd of 300+kg flight animals through a crush cage so small that they can't turn around. Every few cows, there would be one who refused to cooperate. And if a cow decides it's not going to budge then it's very difficult, not to say back breaking, to persuade it otherwise!

All of these things, however, I accepted and even embraced in order to do 'my bit' for the farming community.

You see, tuberculin testing and slaughter of positive animals is the only method of control we have for this terrible disease. TB poses a significant risk to human health and hence can have a massive impact on the economic side of farming as well as on animal welfare. Unpleasant though TB testing was, I took solace in the fact that I was ultimately helping the farmer, the farming industry and the public. So, I felt a real sense of responsibility to conduct the tests properly and thoroughly. I considered that if I missed a 'reactor' amongst the herd, then that could ultimately lead to someone catching TB. Medics still deal with around eight thousand cases of TB each year in humans. Most of these are not due to the bovine form of tuberculosis but it can be transmitted to humans. On the other hand, if I wrongly interpreted a test as positive, then the subsequent losses and movement restrictions would be financially devastating to the farmer.

Quite a few farmers asked me to cut corners during the test, or to 'cheat' for them. I wish to stress here that many farmers were also responsible and helpful and took the test seriously – after all, we had TB in the area – that's why there was so much testing work to be done. But it was always so difficult when a farmer would put pressure on me to falsify results. It shouldn't be difficult – it's quite straightforward – you just don't falsify results! But they could be very persistent and manipulative and often I felt like I was doing something wrong by sticking to the rules and following protocol. And I always wanted to do my best for the farmers I did work for – I wanted to help them too. I just wanted to do it legally!

One such incident was the 'final straw' for my career as a farm vet. I had gone out early one morning to test cattle at Edmunten Farm for Mr Netherhawse. I had been instructed by the 'Ministry' to perform a 'whole herd test' on this particular farm because of its proximity to other farms where TB had been confirmed. So it was particularly important to make sure that we did test every single animal. But near the beginning of the test, seventeen cattle escaped from the gathering pen into a neighbouring pen before I could test them. I asked the farmer to bring them round again so we could run them through the crush to test them before we continued on the next batch of bullocks. It probably would have taken an extra half an hour to round up and test those seventeen animals – a prospect which didn't exactly fill me with glee, but which was necessary in order for me to complete the test. But the farmer refused point blank and told me to "get on with it". At that stage, it would be easy to round up the escaped animals and test them, but if we left it any later, it would have been much more difficult as they would be mixed with other groups of cattle. The farmer told me firmly that we simply wouldn't be testing the escaped animals at all!

It was a difficult situation because I could tell that the farmer was generally very tense and stressed about doing the test. When I started to suggest, as sympathetically as I could that it would be easier to get those animals back sooner rather than later, he lost his temper completely and shouted a tirade of abuse at me, "Whose side are you on?" he demanded. "Them or us?" (meaning the ministry or the farmers, as though there were sides to be taken).

I understood that he wasn't just angry about this one thing that had happened. Like so many other farmers shortly after the foot and mouth outbreak of 2001, he was at the end of his tether. I think that a lot of the farmers I dealt with then suffered from undiagnosed depression and stress related illnesses. The suicide rate amongst farmers is recognised to be high, and even at the best of times, it's a demanding lifestyle and returns can be poor. Many farmers also feel 'trapped' in their work because of family commitments and a lack of alternative skills. I have great sympathy for them. But it's not easy dealing with someone who has lost their temper so completely.

His face turned almost as red as his fiery hair, and he shook with indignance. He shouted at the very top of his voice, and so close to me that his spittle landed on my face. I couldn't move away because he had me cornered in a pen. He pointed his finger threateningly in my face. I don't like confrontation at the best of times, and Mr Netherhawse was so angry that I admit I felt quite terrified. I opened my mouth to try and explain that I simply wanted to do the job properly, that this would benefit him in the long run too. But I struggled to get my words out. He continued to shout at me, saying that I was a 'ministry conspirator' because I never broke the rules in order to help out, and how much I enjoyed making it difficult for them. This couldn't be further from the truth – at the practice, I was the butt of jokes from my colleagues for being overzealous in my efforts to help the farmers I worked with.

Mrs Netherhawse came nervously forward and addressed him with mouse like quietness, "Don't, John, leave her be." She sounded very afraid of him. I looked at her for some help, but she just shook her head and kept her distance. It crossed my mind then, that despite her obvious fear of Mr Netherhawse's temper, she seemed wearily accepting of the situation, as though it were quite normal to see him behaving in this way. When her husband did eventually decide to leave me alone, she implored me, "Don't argue with him, please, don't make him angry," and I could see how very afraid of him she was. It was very sad indeed.

I returned to my car to phone my boss and let him know that I was coming back to the surgery and that I had been unable to complete the test. My boss's reaction gobsmacked me. What a hassle it would cause him to get someone else to do the test! I should have handled the farmer better, or just let the cows go and be done!

As I drove home, still shaking from the ordeal, I suddenly realised that this sort of thing didn't have to be my battle to fight. I could help animals and people just as much in a small animal job, and work much more reasonable hours. Unlike the poor farmer and my boss, I didn't have to shoulder the strain of the current farming situation. As an assistant, I was free to move on from the practice and leave farm work behind me. I knew that no job was perfect and that I would miss 'my cows', and some of the colourful characters of the farming world, but I also knew that my heart was no longer in it. And with that realisation, a huge burden was lifted from me. I didn't have to be 'super vet' any more, wrestling with calving cows, racing around the county after very little sleep, herding wild bullocks, having very little time off and spending most of my time covered in cow muck...phew! And I can quite honestly say that, although I am glad I spent those three and a half years in farm animal practice, I don't regret the decision to move on one bit.

Mhairi Cameron

Drunk and Disorderly

When I went to vet school, I knew the job wasn't going to be easy. I understood I would have to work late nights and early mornings, and spend time outside in the cold, doing heavy, hard work. And I fully expected I would have to deal with owners being less than cooperative as I tried my best to treat their animals. Perhaps I was naïve, but I didn't realise then, just quite how often I would have to deal with people who had much more severe and frightening personal problems.

Now, at the start of these two tales, I would like to tell you that one of my greatest pleasures, and I believe privileges, in life is to be in a position to treat the people I come across in my work with dignity and respect. This is because I believe that people will tend to behave badly because they are suffering in some way. But compassion alone cannot save one from the violent and threatening behaviour of someone under the influence of alcohol or drugs. I have twice been in very real fear of my safety in small animal practice from such individuals, and each time has served as a grim reminder of the depths to which people can fall when suffering from grave personal difficulties.

Drunk and Disorderly 1

Mr Jackson and Ben

It was two-thirty in the morning and I was deeply asleep when the call came in from police control. I let the phone ring a few short moments before I answered, so I could wake up. I always feel a little upset at first when I'm woken suddenly from a deep sleep. The officer requested I attend the scene of a road traffic accident where the dog, a large Lurcher, had been so badly injured that they were unable to move it.

I got dressed and hurried out to my car in the cold winter air carrying my visit box. As I approached the scene of the accident, I saw the flashing lights of an ambulance and a police car, pulled in at the side of the road. Two paramedics and three policemen were crouched down over the dog and there was a figure impatiently pacing up and down beside them, violently waving his arms. I assumed this was the dog's owner. I noted that the paramedics had connected the collapsed dog up to an intravenous (IV) line in his back leg and had placed a nasal oxygen cannula. Actually, it is illegal for anyone who isn't a vet to treat an animal but I understood they were just trying to help (although they were using NHS resources for the dog, which didn't quite seem right either!).

I got out of my car and immediately felt tense because I could see the owner angrily pushing away a policeman who had made an attempt to calm him down. He was shouting hysterically and alternated between anger and utter despair falling to his knees beside his dog and crying at him, "Please, c'mon buddy, c'mon." He kept kissing the dog's snout and he had blood on his face and hands, which I assumed was from the dog.

I could see how distressed this man was, and I was not unsympathetic, but his behaviour was volatile, and I was worried by his anger. I asked him his name as I knelt down beside his dog. A policeman answered. His name was Mr Jackson and the dog was called Ben.

There was blood everywhere and it didn't take me long to discover that we could not help Ben because he had lost all feeling and movement in his back legs. I examined the dog fully, however, for I needed a moment to gather my thoughts. I felt quite nervous under Mr Jackson's glare as he hung over me, shouting, "C'mon, c'mon, do something for God's sake." I noticed as I was examining the dog that I could not find any major wounds. The dog had a broken spine and head and lung injuries, but I could not see where the blood was coming from.

When Mr Jackson had finally stopped shouting, I looked up at him. He realised there was nothing we could do for Ben, I could tell from the way he looked at me, but he wouldn't hear it. He snapped again – there was more shouting and hysterical crying and he refused to let me put Ben to sleep. He became quite abusive. Eventually the policeman stepped in and held Mr Jackson firmly. He struggled and shouted, trying to break free, but the policeman was stronger, and eventually, he gave up and listened to what I was telling him. He nodded to consent to Ben's euthanasia. I used the catheter the paramedic had placed in his leg to inject the pentobarb and at last, Ben was at peace.

Once I was satisfied that Ben was not suffering any more, I looked quizzically at the paramedic and asked him where all of the blood had come from. I was intrigued – perhaps he had seen bleeding from Ben's mouth or nose?

"Oh no," he replied, "it's not from the dog, it's from the owner. The dog bit his hand badly just as we arrived." My initial thought was to see if the owner was OK, but apparently he had refused treatment and there was nothing they could do to help him. Then I felt quite sick to my stomach, as I realised that I hadn't put gloves on before examining Ben. The blood that covered my hands was not the dog's, it was Mr Jackson's and he was drunk and probably under the influence of drugs. Until then, neither myself nor my colleagues routinely wore gloves for examining small animals. I was keen to get home and wash my hands.

But my work for Ben and Mr Jackson wasn't over yet. I assumed that the police would help me lift the 35kg Lurcher into my car so I could take him away for cremation. But when we went to put Ben into my car, Mr Jackson became hysterical again. It was impossible to hear what he was actually saying, because he was slurring his words so badly by then. I looked at the police once more for help. Apparently he wanted to take Ben's body home and it was decided that we should let him do this in order to placate him. I didn't think this was entirely the best idea, but the police assured me it was the only way to deal with Mr Jackson in his current mood (they had obviously dealt with him before).

I firmly stated that I didn't think having Ben's body in his tiny council flat was in the best interests of Mr Jackson, nor his neighbours for that matter. Apart from obvious hygiene issues, there was nowhere to bury him! So I assumed that the police would deal with things from here given that they had made the decision. But no, when I asked if they would take Ben in their police car, they shook their heads, denying responsibility for either the poor dog or Mr Jackson. Apparently they couldn't take an animal in their car, so I would have to take Ben. And then one of them suggested that I (a 27-year-old woman on her own) could take Mr Jackson back home at the same time! At this, I must say I lost my temper although I managed to control myself. I refused point-blank to have Mr Jackson in my car after his previous behaviour. This did not seem safe at all to me. Never mind the fact that I might have to carry Ben's body up several flights of stairs on my own, as Mr Jackson was in no fit state to even walk in a straight line, let alone help me. I was flabbergasted they had even suggested it. But they said they needed to be "getting on now." After a moment, one of the policemen nodded, as though he could see some sense in what I was saying. But I still had to transport Ben in my car back to Mr Jackson's flat, whilst they would take his owner.

The ambulance was called away at this point, leaving Mr Jackson untreated, with an enormous wound to his hand, which was still oozing enough blood to drip regularly onto the ground. I dared to suggest that perhaps they should take him to hospital as he was clearly in no state to be deciding whether or not he needed treatment, but apparently this was not an option.

So the police led our little convoy to Mr Jackson's home in one of the less salubrious areas of town. We arrived at his flat and I carried Ben inside whilst a police officer opened the doors for me. It seemed none of the three officers wanted to get their hands dirty! I was relieved to discover Mr Jackson lived on the ground floor!

From the outside, Mr Jackson's home was an unpleasant, dingy council flat. But when we entered, my jaw dropped, because it was so beautiful! The décor was white, and there were several candelabras dotted about the room. The floor was smart wooden laminate and he had some amazing artwork adorning the walls, including prints of Dali and Picasso. There was a carefully organised bookshelf on the far wall and I couldn't help but notice that he had Dickens, Orwell, Bronte and many other 'classic' authors in neat, alphabetical order. And beside a tiny CD player was a collection of classical music including Bach, Vaughn Williams and Debussy!

Mr Jackson asked me to leave Ben on the (pristine white) sofa, which had been his bed. He didn't care about the blood. He sat down beside Ben and hugged him, kissing his face. I wanted to cry. Suddenly I saw Mr Jackson differently. I think Ben must have been his only companion since his life had been destroyed by alcoholism. Animals don't judge or care what we look like or how we behave. As long as we are kind to them, they will enjoy our companionship and reward us with their affection.

I put my hand on Mr Jackson's shoulder and he looked up at me with drunk, despairing eyes. "Thank you," he mouthed silently and nodded his head as another wave of grief overcame him and he turned back to Ben, to cry once more. I realised that his grief was not just about Ben – it was a whole lot more than that. It was losing the last good thing Mr Jackson had in his life. It was another example of life being unfair to him, of how helpless he was against the tides of existence that move us all. Then, there was so much I wanted to say to him, but there was little point. He was drunk and it would mean nothing – and we all had to go. The police had their patrols to get back to. I had a warm bed and somebody who loved me waiting at home, and a job to do the next day.

There isn't a message or a moral in this story. I just remember that it was emotionally very hard to cope with. I was left wondering who is responsible for the vulnerable adults of the world. Those who, for whatever reason, have never learnt to take care of themselves properly, and who would struggle to seek help because they had lost trust in their fellow man. The police obviously dealt with people like Mr Jackson on a regular basis, and they didn't have the time to spend with people who didn't seem to want help in the first place. It was enough that they had stopped to help with Ben. But I was also left with an overwhelming sense of gratitude for the good things I had in my life.

Mr Jackson phoned me the next day and asked me to come and collect Ben's body. He was less drunk by then, and very apologetic. He carried Ben out to the car for me, still somewhat wobbly on his legs and clearly still devastated at his loss. He thanked me again and I looked at him and nodded. His hand was swollen and distorted from where he had been bitten. I asked him to promise me he would go to the hospital and get it seen to. I wanted to ask him to promise me he would seek help for his alcoholism too, but it wasn't my place to do so.

It would be so much easier to just write people off mentally, and say – 'he was a good for nothing drunk', or 'they were just a bunch of useless junkies'. But I can't do that. I think many of us have experienced times in our lives when all we had to go on was somebody else's trust and belief in us. Our self-doubt may only have lasted a short moment, or it may have continued for many months, but we all require compassion and understanding to help us through these times.

I never saw Mr Jackson again. But I will never forget the bizarre contrast between the thug who threatened and frightened me at the roadside, and the man whose home was that of a sensitive, thoughtful and intelligent human being.

We don't just deal with animals, as vets, we deal with life, in all its guises. And I never stop being amazed and surprised by it, and above all, I never stop learning.

Drunk and Disorderly 2.

The Story of Bruno and Pete

It was 2am in the morning. I had just managed to get back to sleep. But then the phone rang. Again.

It was the owner's landlord, this time, and apparently the only person in the local area who gave a damn about Pete or his dog, Bruno, although I think he was mainly worried about the dog. The police had driven Pete back to his flat above the landlord, who they had informed about Bruno being hit by a car. He 'couldn't sleep' – he'd been worried sick about Bruno. How could anyone be so irresponsible he asked? He waxed on for some time about how much he loved Pete's dog and how he looked after it most of the time because Pete was an alcoholic and a drug addict and wasn't capable. But Bruno – poor Bruno was innocent in all of this.

Poor Bruno indeed. His right tibia was badly fractured, he was pale and shocked, with obvious lung pathology, possibly a diaphragmatic rupture. He may not make it, and even if he did, I had no idea where the funding would come from to repair the leg and diaphragm. And come the morning, they would have to find Bruno a new vet. My boss, kind though he is, was perfectly within his rights to advise the owner that he did not wish to continue Bruno's treatment beyond immediate first aid and pain relief. Even though my boss didn't see Pete's behaviour first hand, the damage in the waiting and consulting rooms was enough to give him grave concerns about the health and safety of his staff in the future. Bruno would stay at the practice overnight for monitoring, but as soon as the owner was compos mentis the next day, Bruno was to be collected and taken straight to a veterinary surgeon in his hometown eight miles away. My boss would not permit Pete on to his premises following his behaviour that night.

The events leading up to Pete's ban on the premises started when the police had called me at 8pm that evening to attend to Bruno, after he had been hit by a car. They mentioned that the owner, Pete, was very drunk, so I told them I was happy to see the dog providing a policeman attended with the owner. They duly arrived at the practice and I could tell immediately that Pete was completely incapable of even basic communication. His behaviour was very unpredictable and he was very, very upset. He paced in and out of the consulting room, interfered with my examination of Bruno and kicked and hit the walls and chairs. Whenever the policeman restrained him to prevent him from doing more damage, he threatened further violence. I shall not pretend to have been brave; I was terrified and also very upset to see someone behaving in this way. He couldn't speak because his words were so slurred and he could not focus on me when I tried to speak to him. He was upset, angry, resentful and most of all, deeply, deeply scared that he was going to lose his dog.

I gave Bruno some pain relief with shaking hands, but it was very difficult to work with the owner's intimidating behaviour. I phoned my boss to come in to give me a hand, and the police officer radioed for some back up.

The police officer and I kept our distance from the owner because he seemed a lot calmer when we left him. I kept ducking in and out of the consult to check both the owner and the dog were OK. Bruno was stable for the time being. The back up arrived and it was agreed they would wait outside in the car unless needed because the owner had such a very serious dislike of the police. The police waited for my boss to arrive, so we could decide the best course of action. The original officer went back into the consulting room and was in there for a few moments. I turned to the back up officers outside and sheepishly said, "I'm scared!" (I wish to mention at this stage that I am a black belt at judo and am usually fairly confident in my abilities to defend myself, but dealing with an intoxicated person who has completely lost their temper is another matter altogether).

The policemen stifled a laugh, "Ho ho, why are you scared?" one of them replied, but at that very moment, the first officer appeared at the door dragging the owner out in handcuffs. Pete was writhing desperately to get free and the two back up officers looked very surprised and leapt up to assist. It took all three men to restrain him and put him into the back of the police van. He shouted and struggled all the way, and once inside the van, he continued to shout and bang angrily on the door for the next 20 minutes solidly. I noticed that the other police officers were now trembling slightly too. I didn't feel quite so sheepish any more!

They were incredibly professional and I must give them my full respect for dealing with situations like this as a routine part of their working life, because it was very unpleasant. As soon as the owner was dragged out, I went straight back in to see Bruno and my boss arrived shortly after to help me treat him.

The following morning, Bruno looked very much better, thank goodness, and an appointment was made for the owner and the owner's landlord to come and collect him. I popped in first thing to check on Bruno, but I was not working that day and was glad not to have to see Pete again after the previous night. Apparently his behaviour was exemplary when my boss firmly advised him that he was not welcome at the practice again.

I called the vet in Pete's hometown to forward the history and to warn them of his behaviour the previous night (although my boss's zero tolerance approach to Pete's behaviour had hopefully been a lesson to him). I spent some time contacting local animal charities and managed to secure funding for further work up on Bruno because I had serious concerns about his welfare. I passed the information on to the referral centre. I was relieved to hear that at 7pm that evening, the owner's landlord had finally taken Bruno to them for further treatment. I had spoken to the landlord earlier that day, because he seemed willing to help and he at least appeared to be a responsible person.

One provision of the funding was that we had agreed with the landlord that he would take over responsibility for Bruno after further treatment. I recommended that an official adoption be done through a local rescue centre. That way Pete would still have access to Bruno, but his landlord would have ultimate responsibility for the dog. In my mind, despite how frightening Pete's behaviour had been, I still wanted to help if I could. If we had taken extreme action to try and prosecute Pete for neglect, and thus confiscate Bruno, I thought it would be the worst thing that could happen to Pete, because he felt like Bruno was his last friend in the world. He was just a young man – perhaps early twenties – and he was known locally by the police and members of the public to suffer from alcoholism and drug addiction. A picture in the local paper of him sprawled on the main road where Bruno was hit by the car was degrading and upsetting to see. It identified Pete by his full name.

But, unfortunately, I was to learn a valuable lesson from Pete and Bruno. At first it seemed that I had done the right thing in organising funding for Bruno's treatment and trying to help. Bruno recovered fully and the referral centre was very pleased with his progress. Pete's landlord was involved in each stage of the treatment, so it looked like he was going to be as responsible as we had hoped. But the best laid plans...

I received a phone call about eight weeks later from a neighbouring practice – Oakdale vets in the next town – saying that Pete and Bruno had been brought in by the police as an emergency and they understood that we had treated him previously. A car had hit Bruno again and the leg, which had been fractured previously and successfully treated, had been fractured once more. We discussed the case and I advised the vet of Bruno's previous problems. I couldn't believe it. I felt so disappointed for Bruno, and so stupid to have been taken in by all of the promises made so passionately by Pete's landlord about taking responsibility for the dog because Pete was unable to do so.

I had to leave Pete and Bruno in the hands of the Oakdale vet that night, I had to let go, knowing that I had done my best to help, but this was one situation, which could not be helped. I find it very difficult in my work at times, because, as vets, we ultimately have responsibility for an animal's welfare and yet there is only so much we can do, both for our patients and their owners.

I happened to cycle past Pete and Bruno a few weeks later and he wasn't using the leg he had fractured at all. The muscle had withered and he carried it limp, scuffing the top of his paw with each step. I could have cried, but there was nothing more I could do.

A few months later, again, I received a phone call from the local dog warden to say that he had picked up a dog he suspected might belong to a client of our practice. It limped very badly on its hind limbs and fitted Bruno's description perfectly. He asked for a contact number for the owner, but we didn't have one. Apparently if an owner was not found within seven days, any stray dogs will be sent to the rescue kennel for rehoming. Bruno was a beautiful big Staffordshire Bull Terrier and I like to think that the warden never did find Pete, and that Bruno was rehomed to a responsible family who loved him as much as Pete did, but who were capable of giving him the care he needed. And perhaps for Pete, losing his beloved Bruno, which must have seemed the worst thing in the world that could happen to him, might even have triggered him to do something about his problems. Of course this is all very unlikely, but it's just my way of coping with some of the tragic stories we come across. And, you know, every now and then, miracles do happen.

Mhairi Cameron

Chapter 8 - Other Stories

A Miracle for Christmas

I have known Alan Scrogham as a client for some time now. He's what I would call a 'Lurcher man'. A man who loves his Lurchers and Whippets. A practical, down to earth chap who would do anything for his dogs. He's a builder by trade, and he looks quite tough, but he's as soft as can be with his dogs. Alan's Whippet, Blue, was a very well behaved boy with a shiny blue-grey coat and impeccable manners. I first met Blue, or Blue's tonsils I should say, when he was booked in to investigate a mild chronic cough. I pulled a massive grass seed out from his left tonsil. It was very satisfying to be able to cure the problem with one flash of my forceps!

Some time later, Mr Scrogham decided that Blue might like a companion so he had planned on getting a pup to rear. But when he visited the breeder, he ended up with Sandy – a one year old Whippet who was thin and looked quite sorry for himself. Blue liked Sandy as soon as they met and the dogs became great friends. Sandy was much less trusting of his new human acquaintances however, and it took a lot of time and reassurance to win his trust.

Saturday the 30th of November was Alan's birthday. Early that evening, Alan and his daughter Kerry were out supporting the local town's Dickensian festival whilst Alan's son-in-law, Tony, decided to deliver Alan's birthday gift which, of all things for a man's 55th birthday present, was a hoover! It was awkward and cumbersome to carry inside and as Tony struggled in with it, Sandy sneaked out through the front door into the garden. Tony panicked and ran over to catch him, but this frightened Sandy and he sprinted out on to the street and down the main road. He was last seen running across the local park by witnesses, but after this there were no further sightings of the dog that evening. Poor Tony felt terrible. He wasn't very experienced with dogs and he hadn't even considered that Sandy might escape and run off when the door was left ajar for a moment. He called Alan, and Alan's brother, Glen, who helped Alan with the dogs. They stopped what they were doing at once and came home to search for Sandy. Kerry visited round local families to spread the word that Sandy was missing and search for information.

Temperatures plummeted below zero that night and the family were concerned about how Sandy – being such a slim Whippet – might cope with the cold. The Scrogham family searched faithfully for Sandy all of that night. They expanded their searches of the area on Sunday and Kerry put up banners and posted leaflets asking for any information on the missing dog. At two-twenty on the Sunday afternoon, Kerry received a phone call from the police to tell her that they'd received reports of a dog, fitting Sandy's description, on a busy dual carriageway about five miles away.

Several motorists had called the police to notify them because he was causing havoc with the traffic. Vehicles seldom drive slower than 70mph on this stretch of road. The police had arrived and managed to chase Sandy off the main carriageway, though they hadn't been able to catch him. Sandy ran off to the bank of the wide river Leven estuary, well known for its dangerous tides and quicksands.

When the police approached him here, thinking they had him cornered, he was so afraid that he jumped into the freezing cold water and swam all the way to the far bank! They decided not to chase him any further once he was away from the main road and no longer a risk to the traffic. They last saw him running off across the fields on the far side of the estuary after his long swim.

The Scroghams headed over to the area, known as Flookburgh, and resumed their search. Alan and Glen searched the fields at Flookburgh whilst Kerry travelled round local settlements to make enquiries and ask the residents to help in finding Sandy. That Sunday night, severe weather warnings were issued and snow fell throughout the Furness area. Monday came and there had been no further sightings of the lost whippet. Alan and Glen took time off work to continue their search. The local community was very supportive and many turned out to help. All day, they all searched the fields, forests and marshes over a wide area. With the last sighting over twenty-four hours ago, Sandy could be anywhere. When it was dark, and the family could do little more for the day, they returned home. But Alan stayed out, saying he would come home later. It was 2am on Tuesday by the time he gave up searching and calling out to Sandy for the day.

By Tuesday, the Scroghams were losing hope of finding Sandy alive. The weather was so severe that local schools were closed and the gritters were working hard to keep the roads safe. But Alan and Glen searched on, refusing to give up.

On Wednesday, there were still no further sightings and Alan dropped Glen and Blue off at the same point across the estuary at Flookburgh. Alan drove off in the opposite direction whilst Glen and Blue set out once more on foot. The weather was grim for Glen and Blue as they expanded their search through the large area of woodland to the marshes on the other side. 'Roudsay woods' has an extensive, complicated path system. Glen walked many miles that day, determined not to give up on finding Sandy. As the light was finally fading, Glen decided it was time to head back home. He called Alan on his mobile, using his last few 'pay as you go' minutes, to tell Alan to come and meet him at the pick up point by the estuary.

Glen felt saddened as he walked toward home on a forest track that was bounded by thick gorse on either side. It was a short time before he realised that Blue was no longer by his side and he turned around to look behind him. It was quite dark by now, but he could see Blue, stood stock still in the middle of the track, staring back at him.

Glen called Blue, feeling weary and hoping to get back to the car before it turned dark. But Blue didn't move, which was very unlike him because he would always return when called. So Glen started back down the track to where Blue stood, and as he approached, Blue turned and ran over to the thick gorse at the side of the track. He sniffed one area in particular and seemed very excited. Glen squinted his eyes to look carefully at where Blue was sniffing and thought he saw a stone deep under the gorse. But he couldn't get any closer from the trackside, so he cut off the track and made his way around the back of the thick undergrowth to get a better look.

Blue was very excited by now and yipped as he followed Glen round. Glen carefully examined along the gorse in the fading light and saw, once more, what he thought was a large, sandy covered stone. As he approached, however, he recognised the little Whippet, collapsed with his front paws over his nose. He feared the worst because Sandy was very still. Glen called out as he approached and Sandy feebly lifted his head up, though he was so weak he couldn't even stand and in four days of extreme weather, he had lost so much weight that he had become emaciated. Blue couldn't leave poor Sandy alone and he kept licking at his snout and yipping excitedly, even as Glen picked Sandy up and zipped him inside his fleece for the walk home.

Glen was desperate to call his brother and tell him the news, but with no credit on his phone, all he could do was hurry back hugging Sandy close to his body to try and keep him warm. Glen feared that they might still be too late to save Sandy. Alan called to see why Glen was so late and he was beside himself when he discovered that Sandy had been found alive. The brothers rushed Sandy to our practice. He was very dehydrated and was suffering from hypothermia; it is unlikely he would have survived another night in the cold. We warmed him and treated him with IV fluids and he responded quickly. We sent him home later that night and the Scroghams treated him like a king!

When I visited the family three days later to take some photographs, I found Alan, Sandy and their cat Billy, who is also great friends with Sandy, curled up on the couch. Sandy is still very underweight, but he's gaining every day. I can tell how delighted Alan is at having both his 'boys' back home safely.

Alan told me that he looks forward to when he can take both dogs to work with him once more and they can all have their usual daily sausage roll at lunchtime. It crossed my mind to advise against daily sausage rolls for Sandy and Blue, but I bit my tongue for now. Mr Scrogham's dogs are two of the best kept dogs I have the pleasure of dealing with and I should think Sandy deserves a few pies after all he's been through this week!

Mhairi Cameron

A Lucky Black Cat

Monday morning and the telephone rang insistently as we opened the surgery door. My wife, more agile than me, made a wild dash to get it before it stopped. The call was indeed an emergency because one of our regular patients, a lovely big black cat, had drenched itself after knocking over a jar of white spirit in the garage. White spirit can cause a nasty burn if left in contact with the skin on any animal but cats are especially vulnerable and also prone to poisoning when they try to lick themselves clean. The owner was rightly alarmed and said he was at the moment shivering; only half dressed at the telephone.

I told him to bring the cat over as quickly as possible but advised him to dress warmly. I had visions of the distraught man shattering the tranquillity of our small village by streaking across the common with only a black cat to preserve his modesty. It was a bitterly cold morning and I thought it might be wise to look up the treatment for frostbite in humans while we waited.

Very shortly, our client arrived at the door (impeccably dressed, I hasten to add) and I could see at a glance that the cat was in serious trouble. Perhaps a third of his body was covered in the chemical and he was yowling continuously in pain.

I lost no time in giving an anaesthetic injection and his agonising cries subsided as he fell into deep sleep. Then, having filled the sink with warm detergent solution, I held his head above the water while my wife gave the body a thorough wash. The washing solution was changed again and again, each time squeezing the moisture out of the fur, "much like rinsing a pair of old woollen socks," my wife said. Any spectator coming on the scene unaware would have thought us a pair of lunatics because after each wash we each sniffed the cat over thoroughly. At last neither of us could detect the faintest whiff of white spirit so we set about drying the cat first in a large bath towel and then letting him recover in a wire basket in front of the electric fire. I examined his mouth because the owner had seen him licking his coat, but his tongue and gums showed no sign of irritation.

By the afternoon the cat was sufficiently bright to return home and the next day when I checked him over I could find nothing wrong other than a minor burn inside one back leg. That healed up nicely after a short course of palliative ointment.

This cat was indeed lucky to have been found and treated so quickly because the mishap could have cost him one, or perhaps all of his nine lives.

Leonard Black

Plastic Surgery on a Mouse

I did not know what a jumping mouse was until I opened the lid of his box and he came hurtling out like the proverbial bat out of hell. Robbie Burns may have called him "a wee sleekit cowrin' beastie" but, under my breath, I called him something quite different as we grovelled behind the boiler trying to recapture him. At last we managed to chase him into a strategically placed gumboot and the next problem was getting him out of it. I shook and rattled the boot until the thoroughly dizzy and terrified little animal came sliding out, probably thinking it was not his lucky day.

Well, it was not indeed and his woebegone owner told me she feared he was badly injured. Having escaped from his cage the mouse had been rescued just in time from the family cat. To be honest, I was not too hopeful because small animals and birds are often so badly shocked by the time they reach the surgery that there is little that can be done for them. However after examination, holding him firmly to prevent a further escape, it seemed that the mouse had a fair chance. An ugly V-shaped piece of skin was flapping loose between his eye and ear but other than that he seemed remarkably strong.

We anaesthetised him right away in a pre-made square plastic container, which was sealed apart from the gas inlet.

As the gas began to flow the mouse sat up, rubbing his nose with his small front paws as if trying to exclude the smell. After a while however he staggered about drunkenly before falling over, fast asleep.

I stretched him out on our operating table, which, relative to his size was several miles to big. Then, having cleaned the wound, my wife held the patient steady while I pulled the flap of skin into place and secured it with half a dozen tiny stitches. The stitches were of the dissolving kind because I did not relish the idea of removing them again. To finish the job I gave him a minute dose of antibiotic before returning him to his cage, which we placed in a warm spot whilst he regained his senses.

The mouse made an excellent recovery with only a slightly distorted eyelid to show for his mishap. His owner told me he continued happily until he died of old age eight months later.

I once watched a human face lift operation and it seemed to me that my present task was little different. However it occurred to me that human surgeons were fortunate to be supported by a specialised team of dedicated assistants and they never need worry about their patients hiding away behind the boiler. Not that I envied them because I am sure that the satisfaction my wife and I derived from our mouse operation could not have been any greater.

Operations on unusual patients are not always successful. We once stitched a deep gash in a hen's breast muscle. The wound healed well but the owner phoned a week later to say I need not take the stitches out because a fox had eaten the patient. That is another complication that human surgeons need not worry about.

Leonard Black

Oh Deer Me!

The local police seemed to have a knack for calling me out at antisocial hours. It was 12am on a cold Saturday in November when they called me out to attend to an injured deer at the roadside. It had been a long day – I'd only finished work at 9pm – and I had just gone to bed.

Even though I care passionately about animal welfare, there are times when one is just so exhausted, especially when doing on call, that one cannot help but feel somewhat bad tempered and resentful at being called out of bed late at night. This was one of those times.

The officer on the phone told me that the deer seemed to be badly injured, but the men at the scene were unable to catch it. This concerned me slightly because I didn't have access to a dart gun. I mentally prepared myself for the possibility that it may be quite unpleasant – perhaps the deer may be running round on a broken leg stump or similar. However, as a vet, I have learned that it is best not to have too many preconceptions about cases and situations because the job constantly surprises me!

As I approached the scene, there were two police cars parked at the side of the road with their lights flashing, and a "CARE – POLICE, SLOW" sign to warn drivers of the consternation ahead. I slowed down and got the fright of my life when a large, burly officer leapt out in front of my car waving his arms in the air. He gesticulated to me to pull into the roadside much further back than the other two cars and approached my window. Before I had a chance to say or do anything, he loudly whispered, "Ssssshhhhh" at me and held his finger up to his lips. I had to conceal a smile because the officer was six foot four and very well built and here he was tip toeing and behaving like a young child on Christmas morning, taking a sneaky look to see if their presents have been 'delivered' yet!

"Okay," I whispered back, wondering what the poor deer would think of the police cars' flashing lights.

The policeman beckoned me to follow him and we crept along a high wall towards a corner where a group of three officers where gathered around shining their torches toward something. As we tiptoed forward, I saw the tiny fallow deer crouched down, looking terrified. I scanned over her limbs, expecting to see some horrific injuries, but the deer looked perfectly healthy to me!

The burly officer who had met me at the roadside bent close to whisper in my ear, "Every time we try to catch her, she runs off, so we've kept her cornered until you got here."

"Oh, er, I see," I said, wondering exactly why they thought I would be any more able to catch a wild and apparently healthy deer any better than the four of them could!

"Where exactly was she injured then?" I asked and the burly officer gesticulated toward her front right leg, which was, like her other legs, poised ready to spring her at least six feet into the air.

I suggested we move back slightly so I could see her move and she trotted up along the wall perfectly. There was nothing wrong with her!

"Erm, well, she looks fine to me," I said. And at this, the little deer leapt up and sprinted past the officers, across the road and off into some gorse on the other side. She was as right as rain, but the officers still chased to try and catch her.

I took some time to explain that there was no way we could get close enough to her to catch her and that the stress of doing so would actually be worse to her than any mild injury she might have sustained. There definitely wasn't any major injury like a fracture, which would have necessitated further intervention. It turned out that the deer had jumped in front of the car and they had stopped in time, but then she ran straight at the car, into the headlights, before running off to the roadside. This suggested that the impact would have been much less than if the car had been moving when she hit it – she had been very lucky this time.

But the police were still very anxious about her welfare and nothing I said could reassure them otherwise, but really, she was fine and there was nothing more I could do, so I took my leave.

As I drove home, my grumpiness and self-pity at having been woken in the small hours was not completely alleviated by the funny side of the situation – seeing the four policemen acting very soft over the little deer. In the light of day and after a good night's sleep, I would much rather be called to see an animal if people are in any doubt at all, but I was so very tired that night that I couldn't help but feel somewhat resentful. I put my foot down on the accelerator as I drove down a long, straight, deserted section of road, going faster than I usually would. I was probably doing about eighty in a sixty limit, I am ashamed to admit.

Suddenly, another car appeared behind me, driving quite aggressively and close to my tail. This did nothing to help my bad mood, and instead of keeping calm and slowing down as the Highway Code recommends, I accelerated even more to try and get away from the other car. The car also speeded up and stayed very close. I was feeling really quite scared by this point and I thought I saw the flash of an arm from the passenger side, waving, which did nothing to reassure me.

I tried a different tactic and put the brakes on, perhaps a little more firmly than I should have done, but I was feeling very angry with this other driver for their predatory behaviour. I thought perhaps they would overtake me once I had slowed, but they stuck close to me (after nearly crashing into my tail when I put the brakes on!!).

Then I got the fright of my life! It was the police and they flashed their lights at me, telling me to pull over. Suddenly I felt sick and my legs went to jelly. Images of losing my driver's licence went through my mind. My job would be very difficult without my driver's licence. Oh no, oh no, oh no, I thought.

I wound down my window as the policeman approached, mentally preparing myself for what was to follow. A likely charge of dangerous driving – and at least several points on my licence for speeding. I felt so scared that I wanted to cry.

It was the burly officer who had amused me so much when he tiptoed and whispered around the deer. The shoe was on the other foot now!

I took a deep breath and looked up at him, but he was smiling from ear to ear and looked delighted.

"We just thought we'd let you know that we saw her again, running up the hillside, and she was fine. She jumped clear over a fence and galloped off."

"Oh. That's good," I said and swallowed obviously, feeling a little shocked. So you're not booking me for speeding then, I thought.

"We just wanted to let you know and to say thank you for all your help."

"Oh, that's no problem, glad she's ok," I said somewhat breathlessly. I wondered if he could see my jugular veins pulsing and the beads of sweat that broke out on my head.

"Drive safely then," he said and gave a friendly tap on the roof of my car. I nodded and smiled, not yet fully recovered from the mental picture of losing my driving licence.

I drove the rest of the way home well within the speed limit and I vowed never to speed again.

I was reminded of something that night which is very important. It is easy for us, as vets, to become so used to dealing with sick animals that it's no big deal for us – it can't be because it is what we do every day. We feel compassion, but the sight of an animal in distress doesn't affect us in the same way as it will affect a member of the public who is not used to dealing with it. So the policemen were very concerned about the deer's welfare in just the same way as I was terrified when they used their lights to pull me over when I was driving. We become accustomed and experienced in our own field of work, and I find it very useful to remember this when I am dealing with my clients, who often feel very stressed by the experience of simply taking their animal to the vet. If I can understand how they might be feeling in just a small way, I can remember to treat them with as much compassion and respect as I would wish to be treated if the shoe was on the other foot.

And of course, most importantly, I was reminded that I shouldn't break the speed limit no matter how desperate I am to get back to my bed!!!

Mhairi Cameron

Lessons in Life

I had been feeling somewhat sorry for myself in January 2009 after splitting up with my long-term boyfriend. In retrospect, I knew it wasn't a healthy relationship for me, but I was besotted with him and found it very hard to come to terms with the break up. We had been living together and I had hoped we would be married and have children. I also found it hard moving to a new lodging and having to cope with the inevitable awkwardness amongst our group of friends as the dust of our parting settled.

I took great solace in my work; I love helping people and animals and I was grateful for the stability it provided in my life. I tried my hardest only to grieve the ended relationship outside of working hours and not to let it affect me at work. But, as everyone who has ever had their 'heart broken' will know, our emotions cannot always be relied upon to cooperate in such matters, and often a tiny thing can occur which triggers a painful memory.

When I met Mrs Piper, I was having a particularly hard day emotionally, although I was enjoying my work and the peace it gave me. As I came to my last morning consult, I suddenly felt close to tears and full of self-pity. I pulled myself together and called Mrs Piper into my consulting room. Her Cairn terrier, Billy, automatically cheered me with his presence. At first, he was timid, but when I crouched down to greet him, his little ears perked up and he was very excited to say hello and have a biscuit. I smiled gratefully, and knowingly, at the good that animals can do for us when we are feeling low.

I looked to the owner as she caught up with Billy and smiled, genuinely now, after Billy had cheered me up. Mrs Piper gave me a disarmingly bright smile back. She looked to be around forty, and very fit. Her hair was neatly tied back in a lovely style, her face was beautifully made up and she was in her gym clothes, ready (as she informed me later) to go for her workout. She was one of those people who oozed positivity from every pore. Everything she said was bright, happy and optimistic.

As we discussed what a lovely dog Billy was, she became even more animated and was carried away singing his praises. When she told me about how much Billy helped her children, she spoke so brightly that I didn't fully appreciate what she was telling me at first. "Ah yes, and Billy's just great with my 19-year-old autistic son – they're the best of friends. We care for him at home and you don't get much help but Billy looks after him, and he's great with my daughter too. She's 14 and she's got Tourette's as well as Down's syndrome and it can be quite difficult to manage sometimes, but Billy really helps me with her."

I looked at Mrs Piper, who was still smiling broadly, and paused for a moment to take on board the extent of her responsibilities at home.

"Gosh, and you care for both of them full time?" I asked. I couldn't begin to imagine the challenges faced in bringing up one let alone two disabled children.

"Oh yes, well you have to," she beamed, "you can't get much help for them. But we do all sorts – when we all go out on the beach, Billy rounds everyone up and keeps us all together."

We chatted about her children for some time – it was my last appointment and I had time to spare, and Mrs Piper remained animated as she talked about the trials and tribulations of her everyday life. Even simple tasks like shopping at the supermarket could be fraught with difficulty. She described her days – how she got up at 6am every morning to get the kids ready, walk the dog and cook breakfast, then going to the gym every day (her 'little escape') and doing the housework and cooking. She was very proud of both her children and loved them dearly.

As she talked, I smiled internally at the gentle nudge I was receiving from life through meeting this amazing lady. I really appreciated the message that Mrs Piper brought me through her happy, non-complaining acceptance of difficult circumstances in her life. I was reminded that being happy isn't necessarily about our external circumstances, but our internal approach to how we deal with them. I still feel sad about the end of my relationship at times; it's all very recent yet. But when I am feeling especially bad, I remember the smile on Mrs Piper's face as she looked so proudly at her Billy and I feel lucky to have a job that allows me to help the animals that, in return, help us all so very much.

Mhairi Cameron

It Happens to the Best of us...

Dianne is one of the most devoted animal lovers I know. She has a paid position with one of our local charity branches for a few hours each week, but the rest of her time she devotes fully to caring for and rehoming unwanted and injured animals. She deals mainly with cats, but also rescues dogs, rabbits, guinea pigs, chinchillas and anything else that might need a helping hand.

Dianne is so experienced in caring for animals that I feel as though I am talking to a fellow vet when I deal with her. She is unassuming and always follows advice and takes appropriate training to perform the tasks required to run a rescue and rehoming centre from her house.

Our local rescue centres are often completely full, and if this is the case then we have no option but to euthanase a perfectly healthy animal because it is unwanted by its owner, or because a new owner cannot be found. I am so grateful for the work that Dianne does taking in animals, microchipping them and getting them neutered before carefully vetted owners officially adopt them. Last summer, we had around thirty unwanted kittens brought into our surgery, or dumped at our door alone (we are one of four veterinary surgeries in the immediate area). If it weren't for Dianne, I would simply have had to euthanase the kittens on their arrival at the practice. There is something fundamentally wrong about putting a young, healthy, well behaved animal to sleep, no matter how 'emotionally tough' one might be.

Dianne is also very active in getting feral and stray cats neutered, another critically important activity. On top of her devotion to animals, she shows great compassion towards people and will go out of her way to help anyone in need. All in all, I admire Dianne and if I can achieve half the good she has done with her life, I shall be very happy indeed.

So, when I received a phone call from Dianne late on a Monday evening, I realised it must be something serious. She sounded very worried and upset. She explained to me that she had been microchipping some kittens which were to be rehomed the following day – something that she is fully trained in and does very competently. The final kitten she chipped, however, had collapsed suddenly and seemed unable to use any of its left hand side. It could not walk and seemed very distressed.

"I think I must have got the chip in its spine," she said, disbelievingly. This seemed so unlikely that I could not believe it until I saw the kitten myself.

I gave the kitten strong pain relief and anti-inflammatory treatment overnight. I thought perhaps the needle that delivers the chip might have done some damage, rather than it being the chip itself, which had actually gone into the kitten's spine. The chances of getting a microchip into a kitten's tiny spine would be low, even if one were trying to do so!

Dianne and I suspected the worst and my heart went out to the little kitten, who remained well behaved and affectionate throughout, despite feeling terrified by the whole ordeal. It conspired that this kitten was one of Dianne's special favourites, which meant a lot because she was not prone to forming strong bonds with any of her wards, because that would make it hard for her to deal with when they were rehomed.

Overnight, I considered the plight of this little kitten. If it was not better come the morning, we had both agreed that euthanasia would be the kindest option, because it would not be a good use of the charity's funding to consider further treatment (which would involve a general anaesthetic to X-ray the kitten's neck and then quite possibly a surgery). Any such decision is hard to make, but I have found it to be true time and again in my work that, when dealing with welfare and charity cases, one must keep emotion firmly out of the equation and deal in practicalities. This way, we are able to make the biggest difference to the largest number of animals possible. These are ruthless decisions to have to make, but they lie on our shoulders as professionals.

However, for some reason I could not let this little kitten go. I felt that we had to try for her, given the terrible circumstances surrounding her paralysis. And also I had to try for Dianne, because it would be very hard to live with if the kitten died as a result of her mistake. Come the morning, I knew that I was going to go ahead with the X-ray and seek some specialist advice on her condition. Neurology, or the study of the brain, spinal cord and nerves, is a very specialist subject, and I was worried that removing a microchip from the spinal canal may be beyond my scope of ability.

The specialist I called was encouraging, and he carefully explained the surgical approach I should make to remove the chip and the various risks of the surgery. On the X-ray, we could clearly see the chip lodged on the left side of the kitten's spinal canal.

I felt very anxious under the watchful eye of my boss, who is very kind, but made no qualms to say that she would simply put the kitten to sleep under these circumstances. I was also worried that I might be doing the wrong thing, and that we might run up a large bill for the charity concerned and end up losing the kitten anyway. But something else told me that I had to try, and I have learnt over time that, after logic and science in veterinary medicine, which must always come first, one can also develop a sense of clinical intuition. I say this tentatively because it flies in the face of science, as we know it at the moment. But for those borderline cases where ethically there isn't a right or a wrong course of action to take, sometimes we must make use of what can only be described as our intuition.

I found the surgery nerve-racking, but, in fact, it was very straightforward! I followed the specialist's advice to the letter and was able to very carefully grasp the chip where it protruded between two cervical spinal vertebrae. The moment when I actually grabbed the chip was the most stressful because, if I had pushed it in only a millimetre, then I could have caused further damage to the kitten's spinal cord.

When we finished stitching up the muscle and skin layers, the nurses and I all heaved a sigh of relief, because the surgery had gone well, and we dared to hope that the kitten might be okay. One of my nurses felt it was safe to name the kitten 'Chippy' (now we felt that she had a better chance of survival) and we gently placed her in a warm kennel to recover.

I was guilty of 'over monitoring' Chippy during her recovery that afternoon, just to make sure she was okay, and I also checked the feeling and use she had of her left fore and hind limbs. It seemed to me that there was already some improvement following the surgery, but the specialist had cautioned me it could be up to three weeks before we could see any difference.

Dianne decided she wanted to take Chippy home with her for the intense aftercare she required and I happily let her do so, knowing that the kitten would be in good hands. I gave a very guarded prognosis, but we were all happy that we had done our best to help Chippy. The rest was up to Mother Nature now.

Only four days later when Dianne took Chippy in for a check up, we all took a sigh of relief because Chippy was improving greatly. She couldn't walk yet, but she had much more movement of her left limbs and was eating and bright. When she came in for her stitches to be removed, Dianne put her on the floor to let me watch her run across the room. I can't say how delighted we both were. She continued to make a steady recovery thereafter and was left with only the slightest weakness of her left forelimb. Soon she was back with the other kittens running and playing and creating havoc in Dianne's house!

I learned so much from little Chippy. Firstly, that absolutely everyone makes mistakes, or, to phrase it better, that things go wrong for even the very best of us. Often I hear people criticised for 'getting it wrong' in our profession, but the truth is that some of these things occur because of a very unlucky set of circumstances. Dianne is dextrous and gentle handed, and she was very unlucky for such a horrific thing to happen. The important thing is that she has continued all the good work she does, because sometimes awful situations such as this can put people off. If it had been me who had placed the microchip into Chippy's spine, I would have been absolutely devastated and questioned myself greatly.

Secondly, I learned to trust my decisions and myself a little better. I knew that I wanted to help Chippy, but I had great doubts over whether I was doing the right thing or not, especially when my experienced boss told me she would not take the same course of action. I think there are times in life when doing the 'right thing' is not easily quantified and we must be strong enough to make our own decisions based on our own set of principles. Sometimes doing the 'right thing' may fly in the face of popular opinion, or we may have to decide on a certain course of action even though somebody will always be unhappy with our decision no matter what.

A lovely end to this tale came when I introduced my Mum to Chippy, who had not yet been rehomed. Dianne said that it would have to be an 'exceedingly special home' that Chippy would go to and such a home had not yet arisen! Well, it was love at first sight when my Mum met this special little kitten and she decided to adopt her officially! She has since renamed her 'Megan' (though to me she will always be Chippy!) and Megan has grown to be a very intelligent and lovely cat, who has little inkling of her previous problems as she climbs the curtains and the Christmas tree and sprints round the house playing!

Mhairi Cameron

Pickle and Gemma

Mrs Parton placed a small cage down on my consulting room table and smiled, looking embarrassed.

"I wouldn't normally do this," she said blushing, "I feel a bit silly really, we've had hamsters for the children for years and we've never had to take them to the vet."

I smiled, trying to look encouraging.

"This is Pickle," she pointed to a very cute Syrian hamster peeping out of the cage bars at me. I could diagnose Pickle's problem immediately from the horrible pink mass that protruded from her rear. Pickle was suffering from a prolapsed intestine, which is a serious complication of severe diarrhoea in tiny rodents. It is a serious condition, which I had never even tried to treat before, due to poor survival rates. Generally the most humane option for Pickle would be euthanasia.

Mrs Parton continued, "It's just that Pickle belongs to my daughter, you see, and my daughter loves her to bits. She wants to be a vet, and she's got cancer." Mrs Parton barely stopped for breath as she explained.

"Ah, I see," I understood immediately.

"I promised I'd bring her here and see if anything could be done." Now Mrs Parton had tears in her eyes. She tried to rush on and tell me about Pickle's condition, but I reached out and touched her arm gently.

"How old is your daughter?" I asked.

"Twelve."

"What's her name?"

"Gemma."

"I'm so sorry to hear that she's unwell."

"Non Hodgkin's Lymphoma. She's had a round of chemo already but it hasn't worked so well. We're just travelling down for radiotherapy today. She just loves Pickle so very much."

I nodded, remembering how much my own pets had meant to me at Gemma's age. I thought of my two hamsters, Cheeky and Fizzy whom I had loved so dearly.

I opened the cage and took Pickle out to examine her. She had developed diarrhoea three days previously and in a hamster, intestinal prolapse is a serious, usually fatal complication of this. Pickle should have looked very unwell, but she was bright as a button and eating normally.

Mrs Parton said, "I would just ask you to put her to sleep and get Gemma another hamster normally, but she'd know it wasn't Pickle. And I promised that if anything could be done, we would do it."

Over my career, I have learned to respect the many differing views that people hold on animals. There are those who would try everything to save an individual animal and not even consider euthanasia when the time seems most appropriate to me, and there are people who would put an animal to sleep as soon as it develops a serious condition, even though it may have several years left to live. I cannot argue with people's ethics, I can only act as their guide and in extreme cases step in more forcefully if I think an animal's welfare is too severely compromised.

Our options for Pickle were euthanasia or to try a surgery to replace the prolapse and place a special suture known as a purse string suture to try and prevent the prolapse from recurring. We discussed the matter for some time, and came to the decision to try the surgery to save Pickle. We both knew that the chances of saving the little hamster were slim, but we felt we had to try.

I admitted Pickle straight away and performed the surgery that morning. The procedure itself was quite simple, but it was incredibly tricky to do on an animal as tiny as Pickle. We had to make and attach a special buster collar round Pickle's neck so that she couldn't reach her stitches because hamsters are very fastidious and will immediately remove any sutures they can reach. Pickle made an unremarkable recovery and Gemma was able to drop by with her mum on their way to the hospital where she was going that week for her radiotherapy.

Gemma and I talked about being a vet, and about Pickle's chances of recovery. She was a lovely, positive girl and she had a full grasp of the situation with Pickle, understanding that Pickles's chances of recovery were still slim, even though the surgery had gone well.

The plan for the week was that I would take Pickle home with me whilst Gemma and Mrs Parton were away. Because of the collar, Pickle needed a lot of help to eat, and I had to devise clever ways of enabling her to eat without being able to raise her front paws to her mouth. I was delighted with Pickle's progress through the week as she adapted to living with the collar on and the prolapse did not recur for the first few days.

I must even go a step further and say that I grew very fond of Pickle that week. She had such a lovely temperament. I would sit with her in the evenings and hand feed her peanuts, which were her favourite. It was such a good reminder to me of the special relationship we can form with even the tiniest of animals.

About five days after the surgery, I spoke with Mrs Parton and was able to report that Pickle was making good progress. Gemma sat beside her Mum during the phone call and I could hear her in the background, delighted at the good news so far. I still warned them that Pickle was by far not out of the woods yet.

On the sixth day after the surgery, I awoke in the morning to discover some tragic news. At first, I thought Pickle was fine, because she looked bright enough as she poked her nose out from underneath her bedding. But when I picked her up to feed her, I discovered that the prolapse had recurred. The sutures that I had so carefully placed had pulled through. This meant only one thing, that the prolapse was irreparable and that we would have to let Pickle go. It was not humane to consider a further surgery.

In my career, I have had to deal with many emotionally challenging situations. In my time as a farm vet, I have had to be hard and sometimes ruthless in my decision-making. But I cried then for poor little Pickle and for Gemma. I had done my best to help, but it was not enough and I couldn't fix Pickle any more than I could fix Gemma. I was reminded that none of us can change the tides of life. All we can do is ride out the waves and do our very best to steer a true course.

I called Mrs Parton first thing that morning to share the bad news and gain permission to put Pickle to sleep – we couldn't let her suffer any more. She was strangely accepting of the situation, but I presume she has had to learn this kind of acceptance whilst dealing with Gemma's cancer. They sent me a bunch of flowers, which was lovely, though somehow it reinforced my helplessness. I wrote Gemma a card saying how sorry we were to lose Pickle, and talking about the entry requirements for vet school, the experience she will need to gain. The day I had met her, she told me "I'm going to be a vet" with such conviction that I had no doubt she would indeed do this. She will make a fantastic vet, and she has taught me a thing or two about life, through her utter acceptance and unerring positivity and self-belief. In two years, she will be able to come and spend some time on work experience at the practice and I shall keep hoping to see her then.

Mhairi Cameron

Chapter 9 – Even More Vets' Funny Stories

Calving Confusion

I had just got back from a calving at 1am one morning and was parked in the drive behind my house getting a few things together. I was tired and it had been a long evening so I had returned from Mr Jones' farm as quickly as I could. I was tired and ready for bed. Suddenly a bright light shone into my face through the window. Thinking I might be about to be attacked and have my window smashed in, I promptly relocked the car and put it into reverse when I noticed my would-be attacker was wearing a vest bearing the word 'HEDDLU' in large white letters.

My very limited Welsh vocabulary includes a random selection of words including 'hello', 'toast', 'lion' and 'police', for which 'heddlu' is the Welsh translation. Looking behind me I saw a police van pulled up in my driveway, which must have followed me in unnoticed. Thank God I realised it was the police and that I hadn't reversed in fear into his parked police car!

I wound the window down a little, "Can I help you officer?"

"Is this your car?" he replied.

"Yes."

"Is this where you live?" he then asked.

"Er … yes," I responded, beginning to wonder if it was April the first.

Mr Policeman continued to question me some more, asking where I had been that night.

"Well I've been to a calving," I replied,

"A what?" he said,

"A calving."

"A what?"

"A CALVING." By this point I was seriously considering the possibility of a practical joke.

This line of questioning continued in the same manner a little longer until the policeman eventually asked, "What do you mean by 'a calving'?"

To which I replied, "Well … it's when a cow needs assistance to deliver a calf. I'm the vet on duty tonight."

"Oh," he said, a look of realisation crossing his face. "I thought you meant a *carving!*" The amount of blood on my face from the cow's afterbirth and foetal fluids must have made the policeman worried I had murdered someone! I think he thought I was telling him I'd carved a person! Apparently the police car had turned at the last mini roundabout near my house to follow me. A few yards later I had turned right into my driveway. The police thought I had quickly turned in to hide from them!

I went into the surgery the next day with a coffee time story to tell of how I got pulled up in my own driveway!

Anonymous

The Cat That Wasn't There!

Hayling Island, on England's south coast, is well known for its association with boating and the majority of the population seems to be involved in some sort of maritime activity. Hence it came of no surprise when the owner of a boat-building yard asked me to visit his indisposed cat. He apologised for the fact that he could not be there himself but said that the foreman would help me in whatever way he could.

Sure enough, the foreman, a most amenable man, seemed well aware of what was expected because as soon as I said that I had come to see the cat he immediately replied, "Oh yes, come this way," and led me into a large shed. There were a few carpenters and painters about, busy on various construction jobs but the floor was fairly open.

We stopped at a clearing and my companion said in a satisfied tone, "Well, there she is". I had a good look around all over the floor but for the life of me, I could not see the animal.

"Er, I can't see it", I stammered. "Where is it?"

The foreman looked at me as if I was slightly retarded and repeated, "There it is, in front of you." Now also slightly upset, I had a very good look but still seeing no cat, again repeated what I had said. This time he made no bones about it as if he realised I was seriously blind, deaf, backward or perhaps all three. He bellowed, separating each word from the next so I could better understand, "There … it … is … right … in … front … of … you."

Now it was my turn to lose patience so, in no uncertain terms, I told him that I was a busy vet with little time to waste and could he please show me the sick cat. At that he dissolved into a fit of laughter and pointed upward. Sure enough, just as he had said, on blocks and towering over me was a great big, newly painted catamaran (boat)!

Leonard Black

Breederisms

Breederisms are all the things breeders say when they bring their bitches and puppies into the surgery. Perhaps this is more entertaining to the working vets out there who hear these comments all the time.

"I'm afraid your pup has an inguinal hernia."

"Oh, it's OK, I go to the other practice down the road for that, it's cheaper."

Thought – why don't you go down the road at 11pm for your bitch Caesar then?

~

"Can you make the clip mark smaller, so you can't tell it's had a hernia op?"

Thought – you're meant to be telling the new owner it's had a hernia repair and we really ought to neuter it so it can't breed the defect on.

~

"I don't see why I should pay more for a bitch Caesar out of hours than during the day."

Thought – would you like to disturb your evening, put down your tea and see you at 7pm?

~

"Yes, I've wormed the pup."

"With what?"

"Chocolate syrup!"

"Perhaps we'll worm it again with Drontal!"

Thought – what the hell is chocolate syrup?

~

"They are 6 weeks old tomorrow."

"Oh, I'm sorry we can't vaccinate them until tomorrow, it's not licensed until 6 weeks in the data sheet."

"OK, they are 6 weeks old today!"

~

"Can you take the blood sample without clipping off any hair – it's a show dog!"

Thought – you try taking a blood sample with the hair on; it's less hygienic and not far short of impossible! It will grow back and surely you're not going to transport and show an ill dog?! Which is more important – the dog's hair or the fact it's not eating?

~

"There's a lump on Gareolisha Penelopee the Second's leg I would like removing – she's a show dog."

"Where? I can't find it."

"Right here, put your fingers on mine."

"But the lump is not much bigger than a pin head, and we'll have to give a general anaesthetic to remove it."

"Well the last dog of mine had a mast cell tumour!" (Mast cell tumour is a very aggressive cancer.) "Can't the boss just do it under a local anaesthetic?!"

~

"Can I have Synulox drops, I took the puppies to the other branch last week?"

"I'll check the notes." Knowing that the client's record had no such consult or sale of Synulox as the computer screen was right in front of me, I rang the other branch who replied that they hadn't seen the client, or the puppies or had handed out any Synulox.

"Oh I paid cash."

Thought – nice try, you can't get them over the counter at the other branch so you thought you'd try us hoping we wouldn't check and even claim you paid cash!

"No, I'm sorry I can't hand them out as I have not seen them, there are no notes on our records so you would have to ask the vet that saw them."

Anonymous

Pet Clientisms

Some of the comments I have heard from pet owners. Very short stories.

"No I don't want the full vaccine – just parvovirus."

"Well it's the same price as the full one and it covers more viruses."

"No, just the parvo. My last dog was allergic to the vaccine and nearly died."

Thought – that was the last dog, why are you leaving this one exposed. Severe vaccinal reactions are rare.

~

"It's ok, she's friendly she doesn't bite."

Growl, snap. "I think we'll muzzle her anyway."

Thought – why do the people who say that the dog doesn't bite have one that always does when it comes to the vet? If they tell you it bites, you put a muzzle on it and no one gets bitten. If they say nothing – the dog is fine. But if they tell you the dog's fine – it's not. They pretend not to see the bite marks in your hand, and if you squeal and make a scene they say, "Oh, it's never done that before!"

~

"My cat's got a cold, can I have some antibiotics?"

"Well we need to see the cat first before we hand them out."

"He's wild, I can't catch him!"

Thought – does the doctor ever just give out antibiotics just because you asked him!?

"You can borrow our cage trap."

~

"I'm afraid your dog has a kidney problem and the kidneys are starting to fail, that's why he's drinking a lot."

"Oh, it's ok, I'm so glad it's not Diabetes, my last dog had Diabetes."

Thought – no it's just going to die of renal failure but as long as it's not Diabetes it doesn't matter!

~

"How long has she been ill for?"

"Oh, only the day before last it started."

Kid "No mummy it started a week last Wednesday!"

Thought – don't you just love kids.

~

The phone rings at 11pm. "My dog's got terrible diarrhoea and I'm extremely worried about him."

"Oh, OK when did it start?"

"Two days ago, but I'm really worried about him, he's had diarrhoea three times this evening."

Thought – if he's been ill for two days why can't we see you during normal working day hours, we could have seen him today or first thing tomorrow but oh no, now you can't sleep on it!

~

6pm. "My dog is really unwell, my husband's eating Maltesers and normally the dog would murder him for a Malteser. I'm really worried about him – do you think it could be the Spot On we put on this afternoon for fleas?"

Thought – I'm examining a dog because it won't eat Maltesers!? I couldn't find a lot wrong with the dog but with some imagination, a back leg muscle felt vaguely hot and the owner did make a comment that the dog had slipped playing ball. I think I treated the owner rather than the pet!

~

1am in the morning. "I've just got in and the dog is making a funny noise."

"What sort of noise is it making?"

"Well it's kind of like a snoring noise."

"What is the dog doing now?"

"It's lying there and its feet are twitching and it's making this noise."

"Is the dog asleep?"

"I think so."

"It sounds like the dog is asleep and it's actually just snoring, the twitching is a sleep cycle, he's probably dreaming, but I can see you at the surgery if you wish."

"Oh, I didn't know dogs could snore. Thanks. Bye."

Thought – are these people drunk when they ring at that time?!

Anonymous

Farmerisms

Some remarks that have been made by farmers when out on visits to see their stock.

"Is the boss off today?"

This is the first comment a farmer makes when you first step out of the car. Most people would say hello but a farmer struggles to hide the disappointment that you are not male, old or the boss!

~

"This is the worst summer we've had."
(Every summer!)

~

"Have you done this before?"

Thought – just because I'm not old and grey!

~

"Cup of tea?"

~

"Will it work?"

~

"OK she's lost both her tags. Let me guess now – 362!"

~

"Have you got a boyfriend?"

It is a known thing that many farmers remain single, so is it any wonder they always ask if you're single. Small animal clients never ask!

~

"Are you from a farming background?"

Thought – is that meant to make a difference to my 5-year vet degree!

~

"I need the test today, I'm selling the cows at the weekend, you see."

Thought – you have 60 days from TB testing during which you could sell your cows (farmers have to test cows before they can move them to a market), you could have done the test 6 weeks ago but now it's an emergency and you want us to squeeze you into our already too busy day!

~

"Have you taken off my discount?" – a comment made when paying for drugs at the surgery.

~

"How much!!"

~

"My neighbour said it was mineral deficiency, so I bought these new blocks, have you heard of it?"

Thought – that's right, your neighbour always knows more than I do, that's why you called me!

~

Two vets arrive on the farm. "Is this costing me double?"

"No, two for the price of one!"

~

"How much for cash?"

Anonymous

Toilet Talk

The yellow Lab jumped about on the table as I palpated her abdomen.

"Yes, definitely uncomfortable in there Mr Innes. I think the best thing to do is get a urine sample and then we can confirm the diagnosis. In the meantime we'll start her on a course of antibiotics."

I tapped the information into the computer and attached the drug label to the box of antibiotic tablets.

"Can you make an appointment for one week's time? Don't forget to bring the sample!"

I handed over a sample pot, and a collector. Mr Innes left the consult room.

Just another routine bladder infection, no stones to feel, but the urine sample would confirm this.

Next week, Mr Innes arrived with Floss and a urine sample. I performed a dipstick test on the sample, as we complained about the rain that had not abated since the last appointment. One of the test strips quickly turned brown, indicating the presence of sugar. When the blood sugar gets too high some of the sugar spills over into the urine when the kidneys filter the blood. Normally sugar is absent from urine.

"There's a lot of sugar in this sample Mr Innes, we'll need to do a blood test for Diabetes! It is quite common in older girls like Floss."

We took the blood sample and packaged it up for the laboratory. The results would confirm if Floss had Diabetes or any other underlying problems.

"Pop that in the post box on your way home, and I'll see you on Thursday."

I arranged a follow-up appointment for three days later, which would be enough time to get the results back.

The results arrived by fax, two days later. My diagnosis was immediately quashed. Perplexed, I telephoned the lab, explained the sugar in the urine and my presumptive diagnosis.

"No, sorry! The results are perfect for this dog, not a hint of disease anywhere."

After speaking to the laboratory, I checked with my boss. He agreed that the most likely diagnosis was Diabetes; he agreed to examine Floss when she came in the next day.

Mr Innes arrived for his appointment with Floss, the enigma dog. I explained the test results, and that my boss would like to examine Floss too – at no extra cost. Mr Innes was very patient and listened intently as we discussed his dog. More blood was taken and sent to the lab, there could be no mix-up this time.

When the fax machine started to print, the boss intercepted the results and he skipped off to his office.

"This is a job for an experienced practitioner, not a junior!" he jibed good-naturedly. I followed him into the office to see his face fall.

"This can't be right, what are we missing?"

The same results! A strange dual sensation; relief and wonder gripped me. I hadn't made a mistake, so what on Earth could be wrong with Floss?

The next day Mr Innes arrived for his follow-up appointment, without Floss.

"Is Floss all right?" I asked nervously.

"Aye, she's grand thank you. All better!"

Mr Innes cleared his throat nervously.

"I'm much better too, thanks to you young man!"

"You must have been very worried about her Mr Innes, I'm glad things have worked out well."

"No, you don't understand son! I couldn't get her to give me a sample, so I brought in one of my own. I didn't think that you'd notice the difference. The doctors have started me on insulin now, and I feel much more like my old self! I can't thank you enough."

With the mystery solved, my fascination with internal medicine had been ignited. Mr Innes is still with us, a bit slower than he used to be and he has a black Labrador called Mac now.

I've never delivered a baby at the side of the road, or saved a choking person on an aeroplane: but I have made a correct diagnosis of Diabetes in a man!

George Grieve

Roland Rat!

Just as I finished the last consult, I was busy typing my notes when I heard a shriek. Rebecca came into the consult room, "Can you please hurry and bring the next client in, there is some commotion going on at the front."

Wondering what all the noise was about, I went to get the next client.

"Who's next please?" There were three or four people in the waiting room, sitting in the corners as far away as possible from a slim woman with long bushy ginger hair. She was sitting right in the middle of the seating arrangement with her legs neatly folded over each other, quite undisturbed by the earlier shriek. The others, however, one of whom was a little flustered and red faced were sitting two or three seats away from her with their pets. Everyone waiting looked towards the ginger-haired woman who got up and walked towards my consult room. I could not see a pet with her but every so often we do a consult without a pet present and have a discussion instead so I kept an open mind, wondering what was in store.

"What can I do for you?" I asked.

To my surprise the woman began fumbling around in her hair, apparently trying to catch something.

"It's Roland," she said "he has a lump on his side."

"Oh," I replied waiting patiently for the animal to make an appearance. I caught the occasional glance of a section of tail and a small nose as the creature darted about through the thick layers of hair which rippled as though in the wind. Once caught, the woman had a difficult task of removing the animal surrounded by a string of tangled hair without resorting to cutting it!

The creature turned out to be one very timid rat, which explained the shriek earlier. Apparently everyone had been waiting calmly when Mrs Jones' dog had barked in the waiting room. This had frightened the little rat who had run across the woman's neck and tried to hide deeper into her hair. This in turn had upset Mrs Williams who was afraid of the long tail that had briefly exposed itself. Many people who are frightened of rats say it is the long hairless tail that they cannot bear to see. The shriek from Mrs Williams had excited the dogs in the consult room who must have thought there was some sort of a chase going on. As a result everyone had shot into opposite corners of the waiting room, trying to regain control of their animals, at which point Rebecca had come in to ask me to please hurry in getting the next client into the room.

Roland the rat had a small tumour growing on his side, which I felt we could easily remove in a surgical operation tomorrow and the consult was short.

She put her rat back in her hair and off she went. It was entertaining to see a loose rat being brought into the surgery and carried in such a vast amount of hair. However I also had visions of her losing the rat outside and us all having to do a rat hunt. It might have jumped out of her hair!

I was unable to remember the client's name let alone pronounce it so I named her Roland Rat. I liked the humour of referring to some of our favourite characters and renowned clients to my colleagues by either a nickname or via the pet itself. I had named one client the Eskimo because he always wore a red or a blue woolly hat and was short and round faced; another client was Victor Meldrew because he looked (and sounded) like Victor Meldrew from 'One Foot in the Grave'. I also had a habit of talking about the pets rather than the clients, for example I would be heard saying, "Pluto rang when I was on call", Pluto being the dog! And "Molly couldn't come in till she'd had a shower!" When in a good mood, I always had a good sense of humour.

Fortunately most clients bring their animals in correct containers or carriers. Anyone carrying a pet in their arms always risks losing it when it sees another species. When I see a carried pet, I always pray they don't let go of it till they are home again as I don't want to have to fix the animal when it gets knocked down on the road outside.

Helen Woodvine

Closing Story – The Second Half of The Beginning or the End?

I hope you have enjoyed reading these stories. It was my aim to gather a selection of stories, written by members of the profession, which fully illustrated all the facets of the life of a working veterinary surgeon.

I have found my first three years in mixed practice to be a roller-coaster of happiness, fear, success and stress. It is an amazing feeling to help a suffering animal and their owner, especially when the client expresses their appreciation, as they frequently do (often with beautifully worded cards, chocolates and flowers to express their thanks). However, on the reverse of this coin (as anyone who works with the public will appreciate) we also have to deal with a lot of negative feedback from the public, often regardless of whether or not we have done anything wrong! I have had to learn that there will always be people who are dissatisfied, though it can still be very difficult not to take complaints to heart. This is especially so as a fairly inexperienced vet, because many people do not want to see a new graduate, preferring to see a more senior colleague with more experience. A surprisingly high proportion of recent graduates will be sued during their first two years in practice, but more often on matters of communication rather than that they have actually done anything clinically wrong. In fact, I would be happy for my pets to see a new graduate vet any day! You will never get an individual so careful and desperate to do a good job than a vet in their first few months of work!

I must admit that I have shed many tears over the past three years. Some days were wonderful and I loved my job, others I would come home at night and cry because I didn't know what else to do, and sometimes the frustration of not being able to do more to help either my patient or their owner, was overwhelming. My colleagues tell me it gets easier with time, but I have always found it difficult performing a distressing consult, such as euthanasia in a short space of time and having to comfort a very distressed owner, and then within the space of one minute to be seeing my next client with a puppy to vaccinate and being expected to be upbeat and chatty. Its quite hard because we are 'on show' to the public for much of our working day, often dealing with many people, whether we are consulting, taking phone calls or doing farm visits, but sometimes I wish I had just fifteen minutes alone to recover from the intense emotional situations we encounter. Many vets are known to be very private individuals, locking themselves away at lunchtime and home time to recuperate after a stressful day.

Physically, large animal or farm work is exhausting – calving a cow can feel like running a marathon and we are often bruised and battered from our efforts (if you ever think of getting into an argument with a cow, dont! The cow will always win, or at least have the last word, or kick, or head butt (and failing that, they can always cover you in muck!). This is not to mention often having to cope on a few hours of sleep after a busy night on call.

For these reasons, I have recently left my full-time work as a mixed veterinary practitioner. I could not seem to be happy living this lifestyle – I am young and just like everyone else, I have many other interests and goals both inside and outside of work which I am desperate to fulfil (even furthering my veterinary qualifications would be incredibly difficult with my current working hours).

I am currently tuberculin testing cattle part time to maintain some income, although financially it is a strain with my university debts. I have often been told by members of the public that "It's all right for you" because they think vets are all wealthy and well paid. However, although we do indeed earn enough to live off from full-time work, many students graduate university with sizeable debts anywhere in the region of £20,000-£50,000+ pounds.

When I first made the decision to leave practice, I counted down the days until I finished. However, as my finishing date approached, I became sad and I also realised how much I would miss my work. For all vets, it's such a large part of who we are. I was pleasantly surprised to hear that many of my small animal clients and farmers were saddened that I was leaving. Even farmers who I had thought did not value me said they were sorry to see me go – which just goes to show that we often don't realise how appreciated we are! But I feel that, for now, I have done the right thing. Some aspects of my job were negatively affecting my confidence and self-esteem and I am all too aware of some of the health problems, which are more common within the profession than amongst the general public. We have a higher than average suicide rate, incidence of mental illnesses and problems such as alcoholism and drug addiction. There are schemes in place to explore why this is the case and to help anyone who may be experiencing difficulties. I felt that it was time for me to take a career break because almost every vet in the country has known someone affected by such difficulties and I didn't want to become another statistic.

Compiling these stories has been a bit of a journey for me, and it has been fascinating to hear about the experiences of other vets. I really hope that the stories give you a true inside picture into the ups and downs of this fascinating profession, and having spent the time to collect these tales, I can now look forward to getting back to work myself, not in the least to collect more tales for your entertainment!

Eve Gurston

Bonus Stories

Long Distance Vet. Part 1

Lambing was going well with my small flock of rare breed sheep. All the ewes and their lambs were healthy and feeding well. I was really pleased as I was a relative beginner this being only my second year owning sheep. My first year had been a steep learning curve as my only experience was visiting friends who were sheep farmers and looking at the sheep in the fields around our smallholding! However my eldest daughter, Jo, was training to be a vet and had lots of experience with sheep as she had helped a local farmer lambing for several years.

My first year lambing had gone really well with no problems whatsoever. Fifteen lambs from ten ewes – brilliant. I had been fully prepared with syringes, stomach tubes, glucose, feeding bottles etc. None of these were needed which was a great relief for me as the thought of stomach tubing a lamb was really scary. All I had done so far was foot trimming and vaccinating. Jo had always been a great help but was now at university over two hundred miles away although I was always on the phone to her. My confidence seemed to disappear when she left for Uni.

Anyway my second year of lambing was going as well as the previous year. I completed a routine check of the ewes and lambs mid afternoon. All appeared well although I did notice one of the twin lambs was asleep. Nothing wrong with that. I moved a couple of ewes and their lambs into the paddock next to the shed watching them for a while. The heads of the ewes went straight down to the spring grass, their lambs sticking close to their sides. Older lambs were jumping on and off straw bales put into the paddock for shelter.

At six o'clock I entered the lambing shed again for another check. Everything was looking good. No newborns this time. Approaching the twins I saw one of them was still sleeping. I checked. The lamb was warm and still breathing but did not move when I touched her. Her brother was happily feeding. I climbed into the pen and picked up the ewe lamb. Her head flopped down. Something was wrong. Panicking I ran indoors to my sister. Fortunately she lives next door as my husband was working away that week.

She agreed something was terribly wrong and got old towels to keep the lamb warm. The kettle was put on so that a hot water bottle could be filled.

Keeping the lamb on my knee I asked my sister to phone Jo at university. I hoped and hoped that she would be in and the phone would be answered. Great. Jo answered. The phone was passed to me and I explained what had happened. I knew the ewe had enough milk as I had expressed some and the lamb's twin brother was doing fine. Jo explained what I needed to do. Do not try to warm the lamb up yet was her first instruction. Aargh! That was just what I was doing with the towels. The towels were quickly removed (apparently if the lamb is warmed up too quickly it can fit and die as a result of using too much sugar – a young lamb has brown fat reserves but after a few hours these reserves are depleted and before warming a hypothermic lamb, an injection of glucose is required to replace the sugar). I put the phone down whilst I collected all the things I needed and my sister held the lamb. Grabbing the phone I redialled Jo's number and she answered straightaway. Exact instructions were given to me. I needed to inject the lamb with glucose. Even though I'd already listened to the instructions, I wanted someone to talk me through it, so my sister took the phone and relayed the information piece by piece. Hold the lamb up by its front legs and against your knees, then take a syringe of the warmed 20% glucose solution and inject it into the lamb's abdomen by placing the needle 1cm to the right and 1cm down from the navel and aiming towards the opposite pelvic bone. Then the lamb can be warmed up.

We laid the lamb on a couple of towels and waited because there was nothing else we could do. I felt bad as I now thought I should have reacted the first time I saw the lamb laid down. I always check now. Within a short space of time the lamb began to lift its head and was soon trying to stand up. I could not believe it. After twenty minutes or so the lamb was back to normal. Miraculous! Immediately I got back on the phone to Jo to let her know the lamb was fine. She suggested I take the lamb back to its mum but keep a careful watch over her. Again she asked if the ewe had enough milk. I said I was sure she had because the other lamb appeared very healthy.

The ewe lamb was put into the pen with her mum and brother and after watching for quite a long time all seemed fine, so I checked all the other sheep and went back to the house for tea. My middle of the night check found everything normal and I went back to bed feeling very happy and so grateful to my daughter.

Awaking quite early the next day I dressed quickly and decided to check the sheep before breakfast. Going from one pen to the next I checked all the sheep and lambs. I reached the twins' pen. Oh no! The ewe lamb was laid flat out. I picked her up and her head flopped over the edge of my hand again so I rushed indoors and my sister rang Jo again. Fortunately we caught her just before she left for lectures. I injected her with more glucose. Jo insisted that there must be a reason and suggested I try the lamb with a bottle of milk, as it was obviously not getting what it needed. The lamb recovered and was put back with its mum.

Back into the house to make up some powdered colostrum. With a bottle of warm milk I went outside to the lambing shed. The ewe lamb was standing – phew. I climbed into the pen, picked up the lamb and gave it the bottle. It sucked and sucked, not coming up once for breath, obviously it was very hungry.

The ewe lamb went from strength to strength although it never grew as big as the other lambs. Problem solved thanks to Jo. The lamb was left with its mum and brother in the pen. As it got stronger I thought it might feed from its mum but it never did and was always eager for the bottle. Perhaps its brother was a bully and never let it suckle from mum, I don't know and suppose I never will.

The family of three were kept in the lambing shed until all the ewes had lambed. I knew the mum now needed to be able to eat grass. I decided to put them on a small paddock, which was overlooked by the kitchen and garden, with another ewe for company. The paddock was also next to the field the rest of the flock were in so they could see the others most of the time also. When the time came to feed the lamb, I wondered if it would still come up to me for its feed. Catching it would not be easy and I did not really want to make a small pen in the paddock. As I climbed the stile, I shouted. The lamb's head shot round to face me and it charged towards me bleating as it came. No problem there then. It came straight for the bottle. This was repeated every time I wanted to feed it even in the dark. The association between people and food became very strong and every time anyone went near the paddock the lamb would bleat and come running to the stile. Hanging washing on the line and mowing the grass would always see the appearance of the lamb accompanied with the familiar bleating. It soon became known as Maasie (maa maa) and would come when its name was called. Maasie is now four years old and has produced healthy lambs of her own.

Thanks to my long distance vet.

A Vet's mother

Long Distance Vet

Part 2 – Maasie

Maasie has now produced two healthy lambs with no apparent difficulty. Checking her teats after the first lamb I found a small lump close to the end of one teat. It did not appear to hurt her. Massaging her udder eventually brought spurts of milk from the side of the teat and not the end. The lamb thrived and so did Maasie but a note was made about the lump.

The following year Maasie gave birth easily to another lamb. The lamb was checked, a male, and was well. Maasie's turn. The lump was still there but again did not seem to hurt her. I could express some milk from one side of the udder but I could not get anything from the one with the lump. The lump was blocking the teat canal, preventing expression of the milk. I decided to leave things as they were but monitor her. The lamb continued to feed well and was growing. I tried to watch the lamb to see if it was feeding from both sides. This was difficult unless you watch all day long. I wasn't sure. I tried expressing milk again but was unsuccessful and was forced to leave it.

Eventually Maasie's udder became noticeably bigger on one side, the lamb was obviously not feeding from both sides. I phoned Jo. Jo was now a fully qualified vet and working at a practice over three hundred miles away. She told me that I needed to express milk from the large udder or mastitis would develop. Jo advised calling a local vet – Sam, if I didn't manage. The udder was now looking bright pink and quite angry so I called the local vet out to examine Maasie. He agreed with Jo and tried to express milk with no success. Sam then tried to make a hole in the end the teat. Not very pleasant for Maasie but she didn't object. Unfortunately this did not work either. Maasie was given a shot of antibiotics and Sam left telling me to keep trying to express milk. He wasn't sure what else he could do and advised culling her after she had raised her lamb.

I was distraught. Maasie, my favourite, was the one sheep I did not want to lose. Soon I was back on the phone to Jo to see if she had any more ideas. She had seen the lump months before but did not know the state of her udder now apart from my description over the phone. The only course of action she could suggest was to cut the lump off her teat. I was appalled; there was no way I could do that. What would happen if she bled too much? How far down would I have to cut? What if I made things worse? Jo apologised but that was all she could suggest, mastitis was becoming a strong possibility and I would probably lose her. Jo told me to use a sharp pair of scissors, cut quickly and cleanly, without hesitation and have antiseptic and a tourniquet ready in case there was a lot of bleeding. What could I use for a tourniquet? I wished Jo were at home. I had complete faith in her and felt sure she would sort things for me.

Pondering for a long time I went inside and put the kettle on for coffee but never managed to make a cup. I pondered some more and walked outside to have another look at Maasie. I did not want to lose Maasie. Action was needed. Convincing myself that I could manage to cut the lump off (or risk losing Maasie) I jumped into the car and drove into town. I searched the shops for a small, sharp pair of scissors. In the third shop I found a couple of pairs that I thought would be sharp enough. I bought them both and returned home.

After disinfecting the scissors I got out a bottle of surgical spirit, some cotton wool and some string (my tourniquet). I went through what I needed to do and then I waited. I decided I needed help, someone to hold Maasie. My sister would be home from work in about an hour. I already had Maasie and her lamb in a small pen in the front paddock. Guess what I did next? Absolutely nothing! I was anxious about what I had to do and could only go through it in my head. I have great respect and admiration for all vets especially my daughter who has helped me so many times over the last six years.

When my sister arrived home, I immediately informed her of my intentions. Willingly she offered to help but made it clear that there was no way she could cut the lump off. Quickly she changed into old clothes whilst I collected my equipment. Very clearly, step-by-step, I explained how I was going to do it. I lined my equipment up on a carrier bag whilst my sister turned Maasie over. Her lamb shot to the other side of the pen. Maasie wriggled but my sister held firm. Using the cotton wool I dabbed the area around the teat with surgical spirit. Holding the scissors in one hand and Maasie's teat in the other I took a deep breath, thinking I've got to do this first time. No messing about. I positioned the scissors carefully and cut hard and firm. A continuous stream of milk shot in an arc skywards. A trickle of blood ran down the udder hardly noticeable. We watched, whilst the milk continued to pour out. We waited but the milk did not stop. There was nothing else I could do so we let Maasie go with the milk still pouring from her. It was now a matter of time and all I could do was to keep checking her.

The udder eventually went back to a normal size. I was so pleased.

That was nearly a year ago and Maasie is fine and hopefully going to give us another healthy lamb this year.

Thanks again to my long distance vet.

A Vet's mother